Control
Your Blood
Pressure

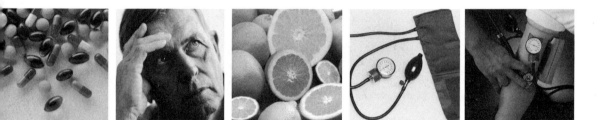

52 Brilliant Ideas

one good idea can change your life

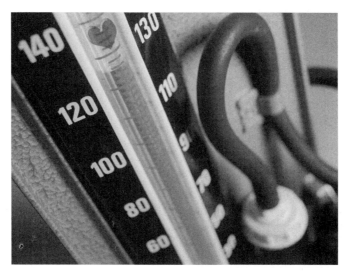

Control Your Blood Pressure

Smart Ways to Get Healthy Where It Counts Most

Rob Hicks, MD

A Perigee Book

A PERIGEE BOOK
Published by the Penguin Group
Penguin Group (USA) Inc.
375 Hudson Street, New York, New York 10014, USA
Penguin Group (Canada), 90 Eglinton Avenue East, Suite 700, Toronto, Ontario M4P 2Y3, Canada
(a division of Pearson Penguin Canada Inc.)
Penguin Books Ltd., 80 Strand, London WC2R 0RL, England
Penguin Group Ireland, 25 St. Stephen's Green, Dublin 2, Ireland (a division of Penguin Books Ltd.)
Penguin Group (Australia), 250 Camberwell Road, Camberwell, Victoria 3124, Australia
(a division of Pearson Australia Group Pty. Ltd.)
Penguin Books India Pvt. Ltd., 11 Community Centre, Panchsheel Park, New Delhi—110 017, India
Penguin Group (NZ), 67 Apollo Drive, Rosedale, North Shore 0632, New Zealand
(a division of Pearson New Zealand Ltd.)
Penguin Books (South Africa) (Pty.) Ltd., 24 Sturdee Avenue, Rosebank, Johannesburg 2196,
South Africa

Penguin Books Ltd., Registered Offices: 80 Strand, London WC2R 0RL, England

While the author has made every effort to provide accurate telephone numbers and Internet addresses at the time of publication, neither the publisher nor the author assumes any responsibility for errors, or for changes that occur after publication. Further, the publisher does not have any control over and does not assume any responsibility for author or third-party websites or their content.

CONTROL YOUR BLOOD PRESSURE

First American edition: May 2008
Originally published in Great Britain in 2005 by The Infinite Ideas Company Limited.

Perigee trade paperback ISBN: 978-0-399-53425-6

PRINTED IN THE UNITED STATES OF AMERICA

10   9   8   7   6   5   4   3   2   1

PUBLISHER'S NOTE: Neither the publisher nor the author is engaged in rendering professional advice or services to the individual reader. The ideas, procedures, and suggestions contained in this book are not intended as a substitute for consulting with your physician. All matters regarding your health require medical supervision. Neither the author nor the publisher shall be liable or responsible for any loss or damage allegedly arising from any information or suggestion in this book.

Most Perigee books are available at special quantity discounts for bulk purchases for sales promotions, premiums, fund-raising, or educational use. Special books, or book excerpts, can also be created to fit specific needs. For details, write: Special Markets, Penguin Group (USA) Inc., 375 Hudson Street, New York, New York 10014.

Brilliant ideas

Brilliant features

Each chapter of this book is designed to provide you with an inspirational idea that you can read quickly and put into practice right away.

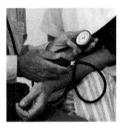

Throughout you'll find four features that will help you to get right to the heart of the idea:

- *Try another idea* If this idea looks like a life-changer then there's no time to lose. *Try another idea* will point you right to a related tip to expand and enhance the first.

- *Here's an idea for you* Give it a try—right here, right now—and get an idea of how well you're doing so far.

- *Defining ideas* Words of wisdom from masters and mistresses of the art, plus some interesting hangers-on.

- *How did it go?* If at first you do succeed try to hide your amazement. If, on the other hand, you don't this is where you'll find a Q and A that highlights common problems and how to get over them.

Introduction

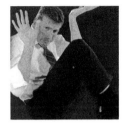

"The only pressure I'm under is the pressure I've put on myself."
MARK MESSIER, ice hockey player

You can't see it and you can't hear it. But it's there, and it has the power
to give you a long life, or a much shorter one.

Blood pressure. We take it for granted. In fact, we don't usually even think about it.
Not until someone offers to check it for us, that is. Or until it's too high and lives up
to its nickname as the silent killer.

Whether you have high blood pressure (medically termed hypertension) or not, you
want to keep your blood pressure at a level where it is unlikely to do you harm. OK,
let's get the scary stuff out of the way. High blood pressure increases the risk of you
suffering a heart attack, heart failure, and stroke. There, I've said it. And this is why
doctors, such as myself, and nurses go on and on about it.

We also go on about it because blood pressure is quite happy to creep up if you let
things slide without you even knowing it. This is why it's recommended that you
have your blood pressure checked from time to time. How often you need to do
this depends on what your doctor advises.

There are lots of simple lifestyle changes that will help you to keep your blood
pressure at a healthy level or to lower it if it's too high. These lifestyle changes may
not work overnight, but given time and your continued efforts they'll help you
succeed in achieving your goal.

Defining idea...

"I got the bill for my surgery. Now I know what those doctors were wearing masks for."
JAMES H. BOREN, humorist

And that's what this book is all about. It's not about scaring you so much that you take up the unhealthiest behaviors you can think of and just wait for the inevitable bang. It's about the principles of blood pressure management and how simple but effective ideas—52 of them to be precise—can help you to be in control of your blood pressure.

Some of the ideas need you to make a little bit of effort, others need no more than you to be willing to give them a try. Many of the ideas may make you think, "Surely this can't make a difference." Once you've tried them you'll see that they can. While trying the different ideas you should have fun. None of them are meant to punish you. Putting the ideas into practice will not leave your pockets empty either, but they may leave you with a smile on your face.

What you do every day has an impact on your health. It either makes it better or it makes it worse. Keeping healthy is actually very simple. Healthy eating, regular exercise, not smoking, not drinking too much alcohol, and keeping stress under control are the basics of good health. On paper it's easy; what is much harder is putting these principles into practice and keeping them up.

This is why making small but effective lifestyle changes works. They are straightforward to do, and they slip easily into everyday life, quickly becoming part of your normal routine. Before long you'll be reaching for some fruit, using the stairs, taking five minutes to relax, and, what's more, you'll be doing all this and more without even having to think about it. As part of the deal it isn't just your blood pressure that will benefit; your overall physical and emotional health will improve, too.

If you're worried that this is a textbook about blood pressure, relax. It's not. And before you ask, the only tests will be those you set yourself. This is a book that I hope offers you practical and commonsense advice about how blood pressure can be kept at a level whereby it will look after you rather than speed up your demise. I have spent many years practicing medicine (yes, I know, soon I'll get it right!) and during that time have seen the damage that uncontrolled high blood pressure can do to the body. I've also learned about what works and what doesn't work to keep blood pressure levels healthy, not just from other doctors but from my patients, who have been kind enough to share their ideas with me. I've also seen the look of relief and, dare I say, pride on the faces of those who've been told that their blood pressure is normal as a result of them putting ideas like these into practice.

I can feel that you're ready to get started so let me leave you with this thought from William Londen:

"To ensure good health: Eat lightly, breathe deeply, live moderately, cultivate cheerfulness, and maintain an interest in life."

Now it's your turn. So off you go, and enjoy.

"There is no point at which you can say, 'Well, I'm successful now. I might as well take a nap.'"
CARRIE FISHER

Defining idea...

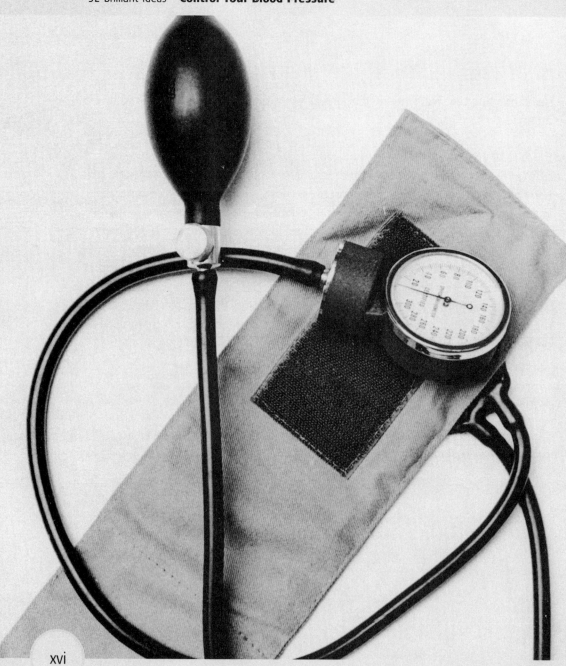

1

Pump up the volume

So you're 120 over 80. Or maybe you're 140 over 90. Be honest, do you really know what that means? Blood pressure explained in human terms...because you're not a number.

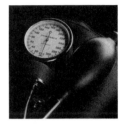

You've had your blood pressure checked. The doctor hummed and said, "That's fine." You took a deep breath and asked, "What is it?" Slowly your doctor raised her head and looked you straight in the eye.

Smiling nervously, you were just about to tell her that it really doesn't matter, feeling you've crossed the line, when she smiled and said, "120 over 80." Sighing you say great, OK, thank you, and leave as quickly as possible.

Two minutes later as you're enjoying the moment the anticlimax hits you head-on. 120 over 80. My blood pressure is 120 over 80. So what? You have no idea what this means. It's another number to add to the list: 20/20 vision, body mass index of 24, a perfect 10, and now 120 over 80.

Here's an idea for you...

Record your blood pressure. If you've had it done recently, then look at the reading in light of your new knowledge. If you haven't had it done recently, have it measured. There's an abundance of places to do this; your doctor, nurse, local pharmacist, gym, or your occupational health department, for example.

The heart is basically a muscle whose job is to pump blood around the body. Blood is pumped from the heart, it travels around the body delivering oxygen and nutrients to the organs of the body, and returns to the heart ready to be pumped back out again. It's like a water pump in a garden fountain. So lesson one: The heart is a muscular pump.

To work, the heart needs a power supply, and this is electrical. So lesson two: The heart is an electrical muscular pump.

An adult has around five liters of blood that circulates around the body approximately once every minute. As the blood passes through your arteries, the force it exerts on the artery walls is your blood pressure.

The top figure, called the *systolic* blood pressure, is the pressure in blood vessels when the heart is pumping blood out. The lower figure, called the *diastolic* pressure, is the pressure in blood vessels when the heart is filling with blood again. The heart contracts, or squeezes, so blood is pushed out into circulation, then it relaxes. So squeeze and relax, squeeze and relax. Imagine squeezing a tube of toothpaste— better still, actually get the tube of toothpaste from the bathroom and squeeze it. As you press you can feel the pressure in the tube increasing, as you relax the tube doesn't bulge as much because the pressure on the inside of the tube is less. You've now completed lesson three: Squeeze and relax.

OK, so you now know what the two blood pressure figures represent. But what you really want to know is what is normal. It's often said that 120 over 80 is the "normal" blood pressure. The reality is that there's a range of readings that will be considered normal, or better still, safe, which is why doctors go on and on about blood pressure. Scotty on the *Enterprise* was right on target when he said, "She's gonna blow, Captain." If your blood pressure becomes too high that's what may happen to you. A whole range of nasties like heart attacks and strokes can cause an early transition from this universe into the next. High blood pressure will cost you financially, too: Insurance premiums, for example, are likely to be higher. Moreover, high blood pressure invariably doesn't cause any symptoms, so the first time people learn they have hypertension is when something does blow, often with tragic consequences. And that's why having it checked is important.

The accumulated wisdom of scientific research has concluded that having a blood pressure reading that is less than 140/90 is desirable. If you have high blood pressure or other medical conditions your doctor will probably have told you that it is desirable for your blood pressure to be even less than this. Here ends lesson four.

When you measure your blood pressure the result may be different from what you expect. Take a look at IDEA 3, *What goes up...*, to find out why this might be.

Try another idea...

"I don't need this pressure on."
SPANDAU BALLET

Defining idea...

3

How did it go?

Q I thought that 100 plus your age was a safe upper blood pressure? Have I been deluding myself?

A *In years gone by when less was known and understood about blood pressure 100 plus your age was accepted as a safe upper limit for systolic pressure. But now we know better. Your blood pressure reading should be less than 140/90.*

Q Should I be more concerned about the upper or lower blood pressure figure?

A *Both are important. In the past it was the lower figure that was believed to be most important. Now it's agreed that whether the top figure or lower figure or both figures are high, treatment to bring these raised readings down to a safe level is a very good idea since doing this will reduce the risk of future health problems such as heart failure, heart attacks, and stroke.*

Q My doctor has told me that my blood pressure reading is good. What do I have to worry about?

A *Those of you whose blood pressure is at a safe level can wipe those grins off your faces. You're not going to get away with doing nothing. You need to maintain your blood pressure at this level. So don't rest on your laurels. Make sure that you keep up what you're doing, but also that you eliminate any risk factors that you still have on your list so in the future you won't be hearing people saying, "There she blows."*

2

Playing doctors and nurses

You don't have to be a doctor to own and use a blood pressure monitor—you can buy your own and pretend you're a star on *ER*.

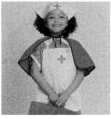

But is that a good idea? And if you are set on buying your own monitor, how do you make sure you get the most from it?

Say good-bye to pumping the bulb while the band tightens around your bicep. Now it's more likely to be the press of a button followed by the sound of humming as the blood pressure cuff inflates around your arm.

Blood pressure monitors, previously the domain of men and women in white coats and uniforms, and of children's doctor's kits, are bringing home the fun of being at the doctor's office. You, too, can now legitimately play at being doctor or nurse, or both, without having to keep an eye on the door.

If it feels like the band around your upper arm is stopping the blood from flowing through it, you're right, it is! The pressure from the inflated cuff around your arm temporarily stops blood flow by putting pressure on the main artery in the arm. As this pressure is released, blood starts to flow again and can be heard through a stethoscope. The reading when blood flow is first heard is called the *systolic* blood

Decide what you want a blood pressure monitor to do for you, what functions you want, how much you can afford, and then go and try some out. Ask your doctor or pharmacist to let you try the one he or she uses. Go along to the store and do some test runs. Think about how you feel measuring your own blood pressure, how user-friendly the machine is. Before buying one, spend some time thinking about if it's really for you or not.

pressure—the upper of the two blood pressure figures. The pressure at which blood flow can no longer be heard is the *diastolic* blood pressure—the lower of the two blood pressure figures. Electronic devices have dispensed with stethoscopes and use a microphone to listen to the blood pulsing through the artery, and provide a digital readout of blood pressure and heart rate, or pulse, too.

Sounds great but before you rush out to buy one, stop and think. Should I have my own?

First of all, why are you thinking about having one? Maybe you are a science fanatic and like to find out about things. Perhaps you love gadgets. Maybe you've been diagnosed with high blood pressure and want to monitor how well you're controlling it. Your doctor may even have suggested that you get one, for your own good or for his! All fine reasons to have your own. Home blood pressure monitors are not a substitute for having your pressure checked by your doctor but they can help you feel more in control. They are especially useful if you suffer from "white-coat hypertension."

Just as blood pressure monitors can help they can also create problems. If you are a worrier, then measuring your own pressure may not be too healthy. How are you going to feel if the reading is high? If this will send you into a panic, it's probably best not to buy one. Would you say that you are very concerned about your health? Others might call you health-obsessed. Blood pressure monitors, like any other health equipment, can take over. It starts with just once a week but before long you're checking it every spare moment of the day and reams of spreadsheets detailing your blood pressure readings accompany you everywhere you go. If this is the case, forget the idea of having your own monitor. It's unlikely to help you.

Now that you're in the mood for playing doctors and nurses, try IDEA 19, *The fat of the land*.

Try another idea...

Next time you have your blood pressure checked, think about how you are feeling, while waiting in the doctor's waiting room, as your blood pressure is being taken, and once you've been given the reading. If you are not due to have it checked or it's difficult for you to go and have it checked at the present time, think about the last time you went for any other test and how you felt, or how you react to results of any kind. I know someone who couldn't open the envelope containing their examination results. They knew that they wanted to know the results, but they felt so anxious that they had to have someone open it and tell them the results. Home blood pressure monitors may not be the best thing if this is what happens to you. But if you feel relaxed and happy, then why not think about having your own?

"What's up, Doc?"
BUGS BUNNY

Defining idea...

7

How did it go?

Q **I'm one of those people who doesn't handle unexpected news too well. But my doctor thinks it's a good idea for me to monitor my blood pressure myself from time to time. Should I spurn his advice or go for it?**

A *This is tricky. If you do decide to get your own monitor, then make sure someone is with you when you check your pressure. Let them be doctor or nurse for you. An alternative is to have your blood pressure checked at your local pharmacy.*

Q **I'm not sure if my monitor is reading accurately. How can I tell?**

A *Get the instruction manual out and check that you are using the monitor correctly. If necessary, charge or change the batteries. If you've done this already, then ask the retailer from whom you purchased it to check it for you. You may need to return it to the manufacturer to be recalibrated. If this is not easy, ask your doctor or nurse whether he or she would mind checking your blood pressure for you with the office equipment and then with your monitor. Comparing the readings will show you whether your monitor is providing an accurate reading.*

Q **I don't want to buy a home blood pressure monitor. What else can I do?**

A *Many gyms have blood pressure monitors for guests to use. You can also have it checked at your local pharmacy or by your occupational health nurse.*

3

What goes up...

May or may not come down. Like the value of investments, blood pressure can go up as well as down. What causes those changes? Which ones should have you worried?

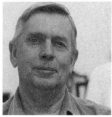

Life is full of highs and lows. We're happy when stocks go up, we're unhappy if they stay down. High fuel prices are bad, low fuel prices are good.

With blood pressure, happiness is a blood pressure that may go up temporarily but spends most of its time out of the danger zone.

Of course blood pressure that is too low isn't desirable either. You've watched the medical dramas on TV and heard the glamorous nurse exclaim, "Pressure's dropping, 80 over 40." The expression on her face and on the faces around her tell you this is not good. In fact you don't need to be told, because one look at the guy on the table says, this really isn't good. But it's high blood pressure that is generally considered to be an everyday problem.

Blood pressure goes up and down throughout the day. If you run up the stairs or run for the bus, your blood pressure goes up. Overnight while you're asleep, it goes

Here's an idea for you...

This coming week record the times when you feel under pressure. Alongside these record what you did to relax. Put a cross by the unhealthy activities (alcohol, sweets, smoking); put a check by the healthy activities (practicing relaxation techniques, eating fruit, exercising). You'll see how you relax and whether your habits could be pushing your blood pressure into the danger zone.

down. This is normal, so relax. These fluctuations are temporary, which makes them fine. Unlike those of the stock market, which although also normal, cause great anxiety.

Whether it's fluctuations of the stock market or something else that's stressing you out, your blood pressure will be moving on up, putting you at risk of moving on out. The meeting with the boss, presentations in public, having the in-laws to stay, all can cause it to rise. As James Bond lay on the table and Goldfinger's laser crept slowly toward his more vital parts, you can bet your bottom dollar his blood pressure was rising.

These increases in blood pressure are good. They are a normal response of the body. They are also temporary, which is important.

This is part of the fight-or-flight response. If you're a hunter-gatherer, this response will enable you to fell that tasty antelope and escape from threatening animals. If your jungle is urban, the same response will help you perform well at work and get out of the way of speeding cars or muggers. Surges of the stress hormone adrenaline charge your body so it's ready for action. Your heart rate increases, your blood pressure goes up in response to this, and more blood rich in oxygen and glucose is delivered to the muscles that are tensed and on standby ready for action, whether that action is to fight or to flee. You're bound to have found yourself in a situation like this. Your heart beat faster, your palms were sweating, mouth like sandpaper, knots in the stomach. Although you wouldn't have known it at the time your blood pressure would have been up, too.

It's when blood pressure is consistently high that things get a little twitchy. At least doctors get twitchy because high blood pressure generally doesn't cause symptoms, so you wouldn't know your blood pressure was high. Not until it was measured, or disaster struck.

You know what behavior puts your blood pressure at risk of escalating upward. Check out IDEA 5, *Risky business*, for the small print on eliminating these high blood pressure risk factors.

Try another idea...

For around nine out of ten people with high blood pressure there is no underlying cause. Years of good, but less than healthy, living would have contributed to the level rising above the 140/90 ceiling. The bottom line: Pressure that is consistently above this level is bad news. Without appropriate intervention there's a risk you are going to crash. Banks adjust their rates to avoid problems, businesses restructure, and if your blood pressure is looking inflated, you have to adjust your risk factors. This means less salt, alcohol, and weight, and more activity, fruit, and vegetables. You can't change who you are, but you can change what you are. And remember, your heart is at risk if you do not keep up with your contributions to a healthy lifestyle.

"Knowing is not enough, you must apply; willing is not enough, you must do."
BRUCE LEE

Defining idea...

Q   I need my daily fix of coffee. Does this raise my blood pressure?

A   *Caffeine can increase blood pressure but the increase is only temporary. Whether heavy caffeine intake increases the risk of a person developing high blood pressure remains hotly debated. People at risk of developing hypertension, or who have hypertension already, may be advised to limit their caffeine intake. However, currently it's believed that drinking two to four cups a day is unlikely to cause problems.*

Q   I'm not convinced that my blood pressure goes up when I'm stressed. How can I prove this?

A   *Next time you feel a little stressed or anxious, slip your arm through the electronic blood pressure cuff and measure your blood pressure. Not if you are in a threatening situation, of course, because you're going to need to get away to safety. Once the stress has passed, check it again. If you don't have your own monitor, you can check your blood pressure at the gym before and just after you have been exercising. This will show you how certain situations push up your blood pressure.*

Q   I've recorded my stress and relaxation moments, and I have more crosses than checks. Help! What should I do?

A   *Don't panic. It's natural to reach for the easy stuff that brings instant reward. We all do it from time to time. The important thing is that you don't reach for the beer, chocolates, or whatever all the time.*

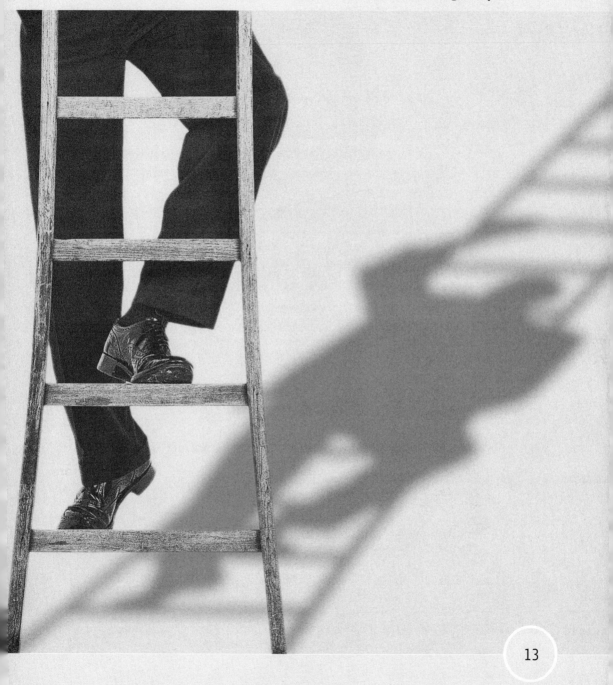

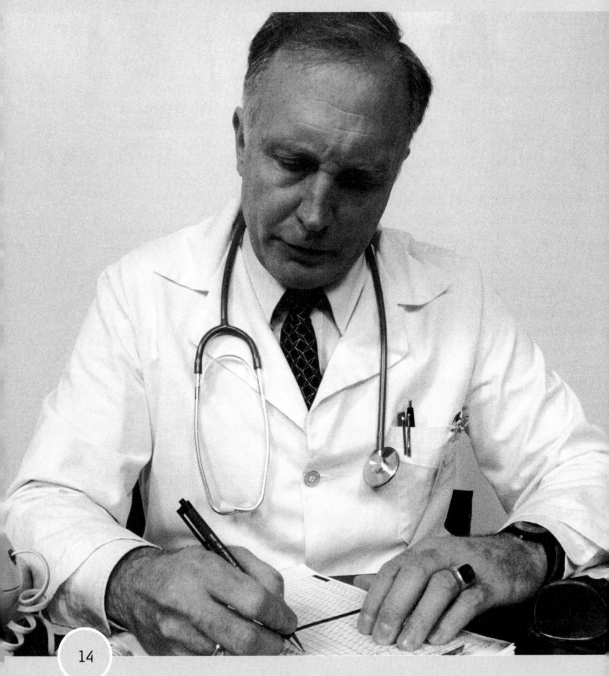

4

Beware the men in white coats

For some of us the mere sight of the doctor is enough to send our blood pressure soaring. So-called white-coat hypertension can tell us a thing or two about the way you work.

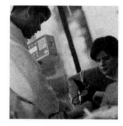

Only the stethoscope trumps the white coat in the game of "spot the doctor." The white coat is a symbol of science and, in particular, of medicine.

Like most things in life the white coat comes with its pros and cons. So beware the person in the white coat—they may want to help you, but they may want something from you, or want to do something to you, too.

You may be one of those people who like your doctors to be wearing a white coat for the simple fact that it helps you identify him or her. These days when someone goes for an appointment they don't always see the same doctor, there's often a new face on the block, and the photo-board introducing you to the different members of the team may be years out of date—the photographs having been cut from the

Have your blood pressure measured by your doctor. A few weeks later have it checked by the nurse. A few weeks after that have it checked at your local pharmacy. If you have a home blood pressure monitor, check your blood pressure with that, too. Try to do these measurements at the same time of day and when your day's activities are likely to be the same. This will give you a good idea of what your true blood pressure is.

graduation yearbook, before the doctor had a chance to don her white coat. Believe it or not, many people feel it's a symbol of compassion and caring, and it gives them confidence so that when the doctor says, "Trust me," they do.

Not everyone relishes seeing a doctor in a white coat though. Some find it sends their blood pressure into hyperspace.

The phenomenon of white-coat hypertension is a real one. Measured anywhere else your blood pressure will be perfectly normal. Sit in front of the doctor in the white coat, however, and it temporarily rockets into outer space. In fact, the doctor doesn't have to be wearing a white coat at all. Just being in the clinic, having your blood pressure measured, will do it. I have a friend who breaks out in a cold sweat at just the smell of a hospital. When someone with white-coat hypertension has their blood pressure monitored over a period of 24 hours, however, their blood pressure is normal.

So in the interest of their patients shouldn't doctors get rid of the white coat? After all, it may mean that the person with white-coat hypertension becomes labeled as having high blood pressure when actually they don't.

This is a real dilemma. You see, the white coat plays many other roles. In addition to identification it also provides deep pockets for equipment and protection from the evil humors that may come a doctor's way—remember how many stains your school lab coat acquired. And, of course, a white coat may hide the doctor's less than fashionable attire—the tweed jacket and wool-knit tie, the sagging cardigan.

However, the white coat is not all good. It can be impractical and uncomfortable to wear, especially when it's returned rigid as a corpse after having been starched to death at the cleaners—yes, white coats do get cleaned from time to time. A stiff white coat may look impressive trailing behind the doctor as he strides confidently around, saving lives like a caped crusader, but try examining a patient in one: It's like wearing a straitjacket.

Fewer doctors now wear white coats anyway, recognizing that the coat may have been a barrier to good communication between a doctor and patient. The absence of a white coat can also make a patient feel more relaxed and so help them, particularly in regard to blood pressure. Medical specialities such as psychiatry, pediatrics, sexual health, and family practice have led the way, their white coats enjoying retirement after years of loyal service. Even the specialists whose white coats regularly came under attack from bodily fluids—surgeons, accident and emergency doctors, for example—who, if not for protection, used the white coat to boost their ego—are now following suit and wearing the more fashionable surgical greens made popular by *ER* and George Clooney. Now if anything is going to raise blood pressure...

It's possible to lower your blood pressure with meditation. Try out IDEA 37, *Let the mood take you,* **before having yours taken.**

Try another idea...

"Always turn a negative situation into a positive situation."
MICHAEL JORDAN

Defining idea...

How did it go?

Q   I wasn't feeling well and went to my doctor who checked my blood pressure. She told me it was high. Should I be worried about this?

A   *Blood pressure is often measured as part of the process of trying to diagnose illness. Under these circumstances it may well be high. Try having your blood pressure checked when you're feeling well again.*

Q   Even when I made a specific appointment to have my blood pressure checked by my doctor it was high. Why?

A   *Have it checked by the nurse. For most people the nurse is a less threatening figure. Most people feel more relaxed talking with a nurse than they do with a doctor. And if you're a uniform fetishist, seek therapy before having your pressure taken by a nurse!*

Q   I tried having my blood pressure checked by the nurse and it was still high. What's my next move?

A   *It may be because your blood pressure actually is high, in which case you should ask your doctor about whether you need treatment. Sometimes people ask to have their blood pressure checked "while I'm here," or the nurse will try to kill two birds with one stone. So if your appointment was actually for a cervical smear test, for example, or vaccinations, then you are likely to be anxious about this, which will increase your blood pressure. If this is the case, have your blood pressure checked after the procedure, when you should be more relaxed.*

5

Risky business

A look at the risk factors and how to cross them off your personal checklist.

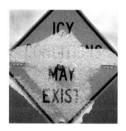

You look both ways and listen for traffic when crossing the street to reduce your risk of ending your days. Are you doing the same for your blood pressure?

You've heard those ads on the radio? Usually they are about investing or spending money in one way or another. You know, the ones where the voice at the end speaks really quickly, and says something about "the value of your investments going down as well as up." Well, health can be a risky business, too. The health equivalent would be "your blood pressure is at risk if you eat too much salt, eat too much fat, eat too much sugar, drink in excess of recommended safe alcohol amounts, spend more time sitting than you do being active, and are overweight." But unlike financial investing, where the greater the risk, the greater the chance of huge profits or huge losses, with blood pressure it's losses you are going to suffer— gains don't figure in the equation.

The good news is that there are plenty of things we can do to reduce those risks, easy things, things that take little of our time or effort and can sometimes be done

Here's an idea for you...

On a piece of paper, into your PDA or computer, or anywhere where you can easily access it, write the following: Eat no more than 6 grams of salt a day; eat five or more portions of fruits and vegetables a day; be active for at least 30 minutes on at least five days a week; drink no more than safe recommended amounts of alcohol; achieve my ideal weight.

Check each one that you are already achieving. Next, choose one that you're not doing but you aim to check off next. That's all you have to do.

in an instant. We can all do them every day. So why don't we? Part of the answer is that while safety steps are drilled into us when we're kids, nobody drills us about blood pressure so it doesn't come automatically. Which means we need a little reminder if we are to remember to get these done and in time make them part of our routine so that they don't need to clog up our to-do list.

I don't know about you but my list of things to do seems to be getting longer. For every item I check off my list, another one, or two, or more appear. Cut grass, review mortgage, exercise, fix leaking showerhead, take over the world—you know the kind of thing. To-do lists often seem to be a life-form in their own right, reproducing and multiplying out of control like a virus. The last thing you want to do is add a few more every day for the sake of your health.

But lists can be satisfying. Not least when you get to strike things off them with a vicious stroke of the pen. In modern life it's as close as we get to putting a hated enemy to the sword. Well, it is in my life anyway. Taking steps to safeguard your health doesn't have to be so tough. Many are no harder than looking left and right when crossing the street. It's true that there is a list of tests and exams you should have regularly but so many steps are simple lifestyle tweaks that will reduce those risk factors for developing high blood pressure. Get into the habit of putting them on your to-do list and enjoy striking them off again. Hopefully they will eventually become as second nature as listening for that thundering juggernaut before stepping off the curb.

Take a look at IDEA 7, *In the back of the net*, to put a check next to the goal you've chosen.

Try another idea...

The kind of things that should figure on your to-do list include avoiding too much salt, eating enough fruits and vegetables, sticking to recommended safe alcohol amounts, avoiding inactivity, and watching your weight. These are all ways to benefit your blood pressure, to keep it at a safe level where it is unlikely to do you any harm.

"The biggest risk in life is to do nothing at all."
ANONYMOUS

Defining idea...

How did it go?

Q   Where else can I note down my goals? I don't always have access to my computer and invariably pieces of paper get lost on my desk. Even scraps of paper in my pocket usually end up going through the wash.

A   *You can put your list anywhere you like, just put it somewhere you are going to see it. You can stick the list on your bulletin board or fridge door if you like. Make lots of copies of your list and put them around the house or your workplace, so that they are there to remind you. Don't put so many up that it deters you—you know how you feel when someone just keeps going on and on about something. Another idea is to arrange the first letters of five words to remind you. Just choose five letters and arrange them into a word so that you remember them. For example, salt, weight, alcohol, fruit, exercise—swafe. It doesn't have to be a real word, just one that you can remember.*

Q   I hate lists. They act as a barrier to me getting anything done. What else can I do?

A   *If you are list intolerant, i.e., lists drive you crazy and nothing on them ever gets done, here's another idea for you. Just pick a risk factor that you need to cross off your list and keep it in mind. Or leave something lying around to remind you. Your running shoes, for example, if it's exercise you're going to tackle, or a tape measure if it's weight. Just don't leave them somewhere where you can't see them or may trip over them.*

6

Chill

Go easy on yourself; sometimes things take a while to fall into place. And when the living is easy, the pressure is off.

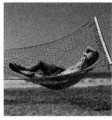

Sometimes it's just difficult to get going, isn't it? You've got something you know you have to do but it feels like you're stuck in cement. Either that or you need a push to get started.

You've been in the situation where you know you have to do something, but you'd rather not. A job interview, writing a report for work, or preparing a presentation, for example. School tests were probably the first time you experienced that feeling of anxiety, of wanting to stay in bed long enough for the task to go away. Even once you've managed to get out of bed, how often have you come up against a wall and not been able to get started? You check your email, make another cup of coffee, every little thing jumps out at you and suddenly takes on a priority of immense proportions. Better file those papers. Can't work in this mess, let's tidy the room before starting. What's that, a special offer from the phone company? Perhaps it would be worthwhile calling them, it would be a shame to miss a good bargain. Let's face it, you're delaying the inevitable, and you know you are.

Here's an idea for you... **Write the risk factor you want to address on a sheet of paper with nothing else on it. Spend around 5 minutes addressing it and then leave it for the day. Tomorrow tackle a little more of it, and so on. After each successful attempt reward yourself. By doing a little toward the task each day your fear will reduce and your confidence will grow.**

Why do you do this? Well, often it's because what you have to do is hard. It may be something you haven't had to do before and you've no idea how to do it and are not confident about how well you will do. You know that the consequences of not getting the job done will be worse than getting on with it, but still everything else, no matter how trivial, needs to be done first. And this is certainly how people feel when, let's say, they need to lose weight or reduce the amount of salt in their diet. It's hard. You've no idea how to go about it; in fact, you would rather bury your head in the sand. Not that that is going to help your blood pressure.

If you don't recognize any of this in yourself, if this sounds foreign to you and you're thinking, "I don't see what the problem is, if there's a job to be done I just do it," then that's great. However, in my experience even those like you have difficulty tackling the high blood pressure risk factors.

If you're still umming and ahhing about which one you are going to tackle first, think about how you've gone about it before. Do you like to get the hardest out of the way first, knowing the rest should be easier, or does it give you more confidence to tackle the easier ones first and gradually build up toward the big one? Be

You don't want to lose your momentum so have a look at IDEA 50, *Oil, water, gas, pressure–check*, to see how to keep things flowing.

Try another idea...

honest with yourself. This is not a test, this is about you putting together your game plan. It's about whatever works for you, whichever way gets the job done. All you have to do is get the ball rolling. Once you do that you'll feel better and more confident and you'll be able to just run with it.

Once the first task is done, those that follow become easier to do because success builds confidence. If you had managed to miss a school test because you were ill—well, you were ill long enough for you to miss the test and then miraculously you were better and wanted to watch TV—what happened afterward? You probably had to take it anyway, while all your friends were playing. You may even have felt bad about missing it. One way or another it would have been better just to take the test as planned. This is why blood pressure risk factors need tackling, because the consequences of leaving them unchecked may leave you grounded, too.

"Each problem that I solved became a rule, which served afterward to solve other problems."
RENÉ DESCARTES

Defining idea...

25

How did it go?

Q   I manage to get one risk factor checked off but then I struggle to get going on the next one. Do you have any tips to maintain my motivation?

A   *Each time you check off one of the risk factors, take a moment to savor how you feel. Remember that feeling as you select the next one to tackle. Write down how you felt at each stage, from butterflies in the stomach to jubilation, to remind and reassure you as you tackle the next one on your list.*

Q   I've tried to tackle my risk factors three times this week but I still can't get started. What else can I try?

A   *The longer you keep trying to tackle this one and the more you find yourself getting nowhere, the more discouraged you are going to be. So you need to pick another risk factor to address and get to work on that one. If you are not careful you'll find yourself not bothering with any of the risk factors you need to address and turning to unhealthy behavior to compensate for how you are feeling. So choose something else and reward yourself for trying anyway. You deserve it.*

Q   I need to lose weight but it's tough. How can I get going?

A   *Losing weight is one of the most difficult risk factors to address. Try choosing a different one for the moment, for example, eating five portions of fruits and vegetables. This should be easier and will help you lose some weight, which in turn will motivate you to address the task of achieving your ideal weight.*

7

In the back of the net

Here's the smarter way to score those blood pressure goals.

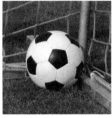

In the game of life, to win we need to score enough goals. One of these is blood pressure that allows us to keep on playing and not get sent off the field.

Life is full of goals. A happy marriage, healthy children, successful career, and good friendships are some of the ones most of us aspire to. There are also the goals that we don't really think about, which you could say we take for granted, such as crossing the road without getting knocked down by a passing car.

Good health is full of goals, too. To be a healthy weight, to eat five portions of fruits and vegetables a day, and to be physically active on a regular basis—these are just a few. Having a blood pressure that facilitates a long and healthy life is a goal set by many doctors and nurses for their patients. Your doctor may have already set this one for you.

Achieving a goal makes us feel good. We are proud to have done what we set out to do. You only have to look at the delight on a soccer player's face when the ball hits the back of the net to see how good it feels.

Here's an idea for you...

Set yourself a goal that will help toward you lifting the trophy—a healthy blood pressure. Start by choosing something easy and use the SMARTER system described here. Try to achieve this by the end of the next week. The more goals you score the more positive you will be about tackling the next one.

So how do you go about making sure it happens?

You're more likely to achieve the lifestyle changes you need to make for your blood pressure to remain healthy if you have good goal-setting skills. And for this you need to get smart, or better still, get SMARTER.

First of all, the goal has to be *Specific* to you, something that you want to achieve. That's easy. You want to have a healthy blood pressure. Next, your goal needs to be *Measurable*—so your blood pressure needs to remain at, or return to, the level recommended by your doctor, which will be below 140/90.

The goal must be *Achievable*. There's little point in trying to become captain of the women's swim team if you're a man. And the goal must be *Relevant* to you, otherwise it's going to feel like you are being forced to climb a mountain. So, for example, do you want to control your blood pressure so you live longer and see your grandchildren grow up, or do you really want to control it to get your doctor off your case? Perhaps the mere mention of having to take medication is enough of a reason for you. You may have heard that your insurance premiums will soar if your blood pressure stays or becomes high.

There's a famous slogan that I first saw on a friend's coffee mug—"a round toit." It's a phrase we all use from time to time when we don't particularly want to do something. Yes dear, I'll get "a round toit." When? Sometime soon. Sometime never, more like. So goals have to be *Time* specific and must have a deadline.

Possibly the most important factor is that pushing toward the goal line must be *Enjoyable*. This is really what makes the difference between success and failure. If the route to the goal is paved with obstacles, and one of those obstacles is that you absolutely loathe having to do something, then let's be honest, you're not going to make it, are you?

And it's got to be *Realistic*, which simply reinforces that the goal must be relevant and achievable for you, not someone else who wants you to achieve the goal.

Let's say, for example, that your first goal is to eat five portions of fruits and vegetables each day. This is specific to you. It's also measurable, achievable, and relevant. It's certainly enjoyable and eminently realistic. Once you've achieved one goal, you can tackle another in the same way.

If you'd like to make scoring goals even easier, take a look at IDEA 8, *Two's company, three's not always a crowd.*

Try another idea...

"Old habits cannot be thrown out the upstairs window. They must be coaxed down the stairs one step at a time."
MARK TWAIN

Defining idea...

"Always bear in mind that your own resolution to succeed is more important than any other."
ABRAHAM LINCOLN

Defining idea...

29

How did it go?

Q **Lowering my blood pressure doesn't really rock my world. It's what my doctor wants. But why should I do what she tells me?**

A *This is why it's vital to make the goal relevant and attractive to you. With smoking, the goal is often saving money or to protect your children. With losing weight, the goal for you may be being able to wear a smaller dress size, or not being embarrassed by your gut poolside. When you achieve your goal the side effect is that your doctor's goal for you, lowering your blood pressure, is also likely to be achieved. It's a win–win situation.*

Q **I didn't achieve the goal within the time frame. What should I do now?**

A *Perhaps you were being too optimistic or had chosen a goal that's not achievable at the present time. This is why people often don't succeed if they decide to get fit on vacation or during the holidays. Start when your routine is normal—don't start your healthy eating goal the day of a friend's dinner party, for example. Moreover, start when you are ready, not when someone tells you to.*

Q **I keep getting tripped up by my old habits. How can I ditch these?**

A *Having a game plan is key. Plan what you will do when you feel the urge to eat chocolate or are faced with a lighting-up situation. Address the barriers that have stopped you from succeeding previously before you try again. For example, if you're trying to eat more fruit but it's cookies you always have on your desk, move the cookies and put fruit there instead.*

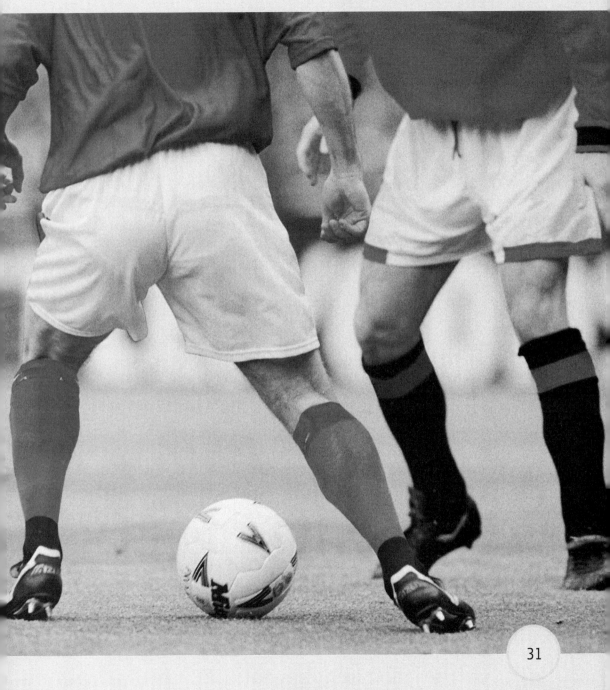

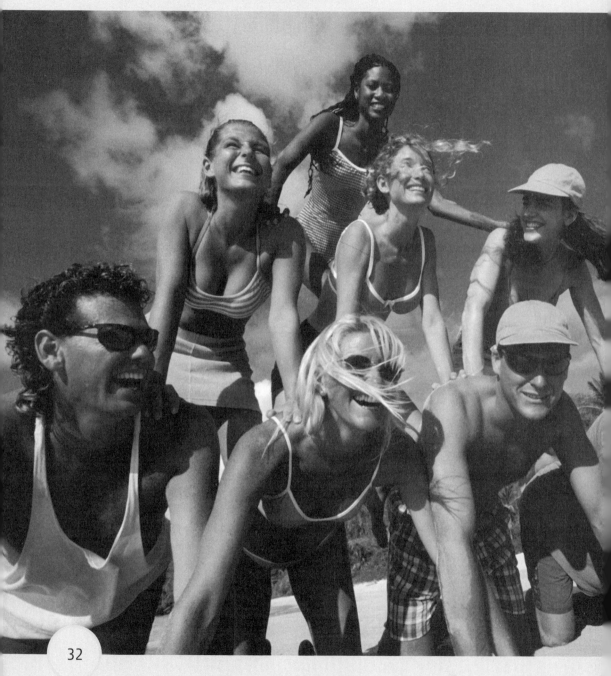

8

Two's company, three's not always a crowd

Too many cooks may not spoil the broth, because many hands can make light work of blood pressure.

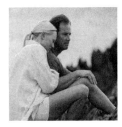

You have to do stuff around the house...home repair, housework, weeding the garden. Having someone to help you makes doing these things easier, doesn't it?

Well, usually it does. But if that someone is your delightful son or daughter who, having seen you weeding, is now pulling out the plants you've just settled into their new home, it may be a completely different story.

These tasks may not be what you want to spend your time doing but they need to be done and, to be honest, they're usually routine and straightforward.

Attacking a problem together, with others, has many benefits. Hanging curtains, even putting linens onto a bed, is easier when there are two of you.

Here's an idea for you...

Find a friend who also needs or wants to get fit. Decide together what exercise you'd both like to do. Each time you do it you award yourself a point. The one who scores the least at the end of the week pays for an evening out—a meal, a movie, or the beer tab. This isn't a particularly serious challenge, but it's fun and motivating. It's up to you what level of challenge you set and what your reward is.

I'm not talking necessarily about breaking records here, although if that's your goal, then go for it. I'm talking about simply achieving the lifestyle changes that you know or have been advised will help look after your blood pressure. Take exercising regularly, for instance. If you've never done this before, or you've gotten out of the habit, then it's likely to be difficult to get going again. Our lives are busy. Exercise is just one thing on a very long list, and with so many other things to do there just may not be enough time to fit exercise into the schedule. Sometimes it may feel that your doctor, nurse, or even your mate is like the helpful child when they're telling you to do more exercise, to stop smoking, and to lose some weight. They want to help you but their constant encouragement is actually having the opposite effect and is pushing you toward the bar rather than the gym.

Generally speaking, a task is less daunting, and dare I say more fun, when you're not alone. If you've ever had to do a simple home repair but have been overwhelmed by the instructions or the mountain of goods and tools at the store, then you'll know what I mean. This is one of the reasons why weight-loss programs and quit-smoking programs that are run as groups work well. The environment is supportive and conducive to taking part; you're not alone in the battle. The group not only provides the support, it provides the motivation and the challenge, too. And there's the guilt thing: You don't want to let them down.

Getting it together is a great start. Have a look at IDEA 11, *On your bike*, to see how to keep it up.

Try another idea…

If you're someone who is disciplined and gets everything done, then well done, keep it up. If, however, you're struggling, then phone a friend. You see, often it's difficult to take that first step, and even then once you're on your way, it's tough keeping yourself motivated. Some people are just not up for any challenge. It's not the way they work. Doing some exercise on a regular basis is one of the more difficult blood-pressure-benefiting lifestyle changes you can make. This is why having a sparring partner can help. You're not going to be trying to punch each other's lights out (not unless that's the activity you've both decided to do). You are simply going to make use of each other to get over the hurdles, such as shyness, inexperience, a lack of confidence in new places—the things that may have hindered you before. Moreover, since you won't want to let your friend down, automatically you'll have established a routine of exercising regularly.

"Good friends are good for your health."
IRWIN SARASON, psychologist

Defining idea…

35

How did it go?

Q **My friend and I did well for the first few weeks but then we seemed to peter out. Now we hardly go to the gym at all. How can we get back into the swing of it?**

A *Don't panic, this is a common problem. You've become bored. You need to find a different activity, or set yourselves a different challenge, or do both. It may mean asking a different friend to get involved if you are still motivated but it's your friend who has lost interest. If your friend was always footing the bill each week because you were always winning, then perhaps think about a different reward system that will encourage him or her to become motivated again.*

Q **My friend keeps pulling out. If it's not because of work it's a problem with the children. How should I deal with this?**

A *Your friend may not have the time at the moment, and if this is the case that's tough. The timing you both chose may no longer be convenient, so think about changing it. Perhaps your friend doesn't particularly enjoy the activity? In which case suggest changing it. You may have to ask someone else because the reality is it sometimes is very difficult to commit. That's just life!*

Q **I wanted to play badminton but it wasn't long before my friend lost interest. Now I'm losing interest, too. How can I get my enthusiasm back?**

A *Ask at the center where you were playing if there is a club. If so, you could join and then you'll always have someone to play against. If you ask another friend, think about choosing a different activity. Something that you can do together but that can also be done on your own, such as an exercise class, the gym, or swimming.*

9

Active hedonism

The sheer pleasure of staying in shape doesn't have to stop once you're out of the 18 to 30 age bracket. Let's find out how to keep those endorphins flowing while having some fun.

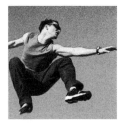

So how did you feel when your doctor said that you should exercise more? I doubt that you felt pleased. Your heart probably sank, which ironically it may do if you don't follow the advice.

Personally, I don't like the word "exercise." It tends to have negative associations for many people. Going to the gym, running marathons, aerobics classes. Immediately you think: How am I going to find the time? It's going to cost me money. I don't even like exercise. In fact, I would not be surprised if when your doctor suggested that you do more exercise your response was "But I don't like the gym."

So I think *activity* is a better word. Not only is it associated with things you are probably already doing, but it can also be associated with aspects of your daily life. It shouldn't mean that you have to fly over hurdles before you achieve your daily activity quota. If you like going to the gym or taking part in aerobics, body

Here's an idea for you... **For each of the next seven days, write down an activity you will enjoy doing. Put the list somewhere you can easily see it—on the fridge, in your PDA, on the bathroom mirror—to remind you. Each day do the activity. By choosing how you are active you have taken control, and by wanting to do it you will actually make it happen.**

sculpture, or kickboxing classes, then that's great. Really, it is. Because you enjoy it.

If you're someone who has trouble dragging your butt out of bed in the morning and going to work—you know, the alarm going off is just a cue to hit that snooze button—I'd suggest that although this might be you on a workday, it's not you every day. If you need to be up early to catch your vacation flight, then you'll have no trouble getting up. Even if you still like to stay in bed on the first day of your vacation, it's still easier to get up than if you were going to work.

The reason is simple. You are looking forward to going on vacation or having a day out with friends, so the barriers that prevented you from getting out of bed in time to catch the bus or train to work have disappeared. You have an easy run. Remember when you were in school and you had to do your homework, that feeling of not wanting to do it? You don't? Of course you do! You knew that you were going to have to do it one way or another but if it was a subject you enjoyed, especially if you were confident about being able to complete the homework without much effort, it was much easier to get going. In fact, afterward you not only felt relieved that it was done and out of the way, you felt good.

Think back to activities that you used to do in school or college, that you enjoyed doing but for one reason or another you no longer do. Maybe you used to play rugby or volleyball. In college you may have played hockey or rowed. Think back to how much you enjoyed taking

OK, so now you're getting there. Have a look at IDEA 42, *Hairbrush idol*, to see how Madonna, Justin, and Beyoncé can keep you in the groove.

Try another idea...

part. Why did you stop? Was it because you and your teammates all went your separate ways? Or did college parties start to take priority? There's a good chance that work or children arrived and took precedence. You didn't stop because you no longer enjoyed it, you stopped because something got in the way. So what's stopping you from taking up the activity again? Probably nothing, so go on, give it another try. In fact, you can go and do anything active that you enjoy. It really can be anything you choose. Go for a run, ride your bike, dance to the music on the radio, throw a ball against the wall, do some gardening, anything at all, but in the words of a well-known sports attire company—just do it.

"The physically fit can enjoy their vices."
LORD PERCIVAL, military commander

Defining idea...

How did it go?

Q I used to play hockey at school and I'd love to play again but I'm not fit enough...and aren't I too old anyway?

A *You're making excuses and letting these barriers get in the way. Sure, you are older and you may not be as fit as you were when you were at school, but if you start playing again you'll soon get fitter. Many clubs have veteran's teams, and by veterans they often mean for people over thirty or forty years old. These teams are full of people like you who said the same things to begin with. The pace of the game may be a little slower but they are still getting as much pleasure from playing as they ever did.*

Q I think that I'd like to try a body combat class but I've never done it before and don't know how I'll do. How do I get started?

A *You never know until you try it. Many gyms and sports centers offer introduction classes precisely for this reason. It offers you the chance to try it out to see how you like it. Usually all of the participants are in the same boat so there's no need to feel shy about going. You could try lots of different introductory classes. This way you will get a taste of those offered and find out which ones you really enjoy—and are therefore most likely to stick with.*

10

Pump that body

The thought of Lycra-clad rippling bodies may send you reaching for the doughnuts. But the gym offers so much more than just firm butts and abs. Take a look.

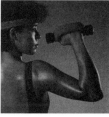

If you're a gym regular, then you'll know the true joy of a good workout. You feel pumped, the endorphins are flowing, and your whole body feels great.

You either love the gym or you loathe it. There's not much in-between. So what's the appeal? Well, to start with, if you work and the walls of your home and your office are the only places you see during the week, then just visiting the gym is an outing and offers the chance to meet people. You can ogle the beautiful people (discreetly, of course!) and that includes looking at yourself in the mirror for more than a few minutes without being labeled a poser. You can watch wall-to-wall TV, too. I remember being at the gym on a World Cup match day. I'd never seen so many people there. Pumping away on the treadmill or the cross-trainer while watching the match—there was no better way to feel like you were part of the game.

Here's an idea for you...

Your optimum training zone is between 70–90 percent of your maximum heart rate (MHR). To find it subtract your age in years from 220 to get your MHR, then multiply your MHR by, let's say, 0.8 (80 percent). This is the maximum number of heartbeats per minute you should have during your workout to efficiently burn fat.

It's easy to forget that the main purpose of the gym is to exercise, which helps keep your blood pressure healthy. In fact, if you walk or cycle to the gym and back you'll have probably done enough exercise without even going into the gym itself. You can't be blamed for forgetting the gym is a place of exercise. After all, you enter and there's the coffee bar with its range of allegedly healthy snacks on the counter. It's like the souvenir shop at a tourist trap. You are supposed to visit it on your way out but it's often the first, and sometimes the only, place you get to spend time in.

OK. Time to be serious—difficult when the mind is full of Lycra, I know. One of the main benefits of the gym is that there are usually a variety of exercise options available. Studio-based aerobics classes, circuit training, free and fixed resistance machine weights, rowing machines, exercise bikes, treadmills, exercise balls, to name but a few. So there really is something to suit everyone. Strength, cardiovascular fitness, flexibility, body shape, and, of course, weight can all be improved.

If you get out of breath when you are being active or exercising, then you are cardio-training, or doing aerobic exercise. Your heart and lungs will be working harder and your fitness will be improving. Your pulse (or heart rate) will increase. If you haven't measured your pulse before, this is how you measure it at your wrist: Using the pad of your fingertips, not your thumb, follow the line of your thumb and place two fingers—your index and middle fingers—onto your arm around an inch past the wrist crease. Count the pulse for 15 seconds and then multiply this figure by 4. This is your pulse, or heart rate per minute. It takes a little practice but you'll soon get the hang of it. If it's just not happening for you, you could buy a heart rate monitor that will do the job. Many exercise machines now have a heart rate monitor built in to them, so you can always take the reading from these.

You should have stretched while at the gym but stretching offers much more than meets the eye. Take a peek at IDEA 44, *The joy of stretch*.

Try another idea...

While exercising you should be burning fat, too, which is, after all, what you want to be losing. To burn fat efficiently you need to be exercising in your optimum training zone. No, this isn't the part of the gym where you feel happiest, like the bar. It's the heart rate you need to be working at if you want to burn fat efficiently and therefore lose weight.

"*Training gives us an outlet for suppressed energies created by stress and thus tones the spirit just as exercise conditions the body.*"
ARNOLD SCHWARZENEGGER

Defining idea...

How did it go?

Q **I really want to go to the gym. I've paid my membership, but I keep finding excuses to skip it. How can I get motivated?**

A   *Ask yourself what is preventing you from going. Is it that you feel shy or embarrassed? Think about going with a friend—safety in numbers and all that. Gyms, like anywhere new, can be quite daunting if you've never been before, especially if you haven't yet achieved that pin-up look. If it's because you don't believe you have the time, try going when you would normally be sitting in front of the TV at home. You can still watch your chosen program—TV news, MTV, your favorite sitcom—but you'll be exercising at the same time. Just make sure that you put some effort into the exercise, don't be an "exercise-bike potato."*

Q **I can't even turn on the DVD player. How will I know what to do when I get there?**

A   *First of all, you don't have to use the equipment, you can do an aerobics class. There are often introductory classes for first timers. Nine times out of ten, gym users are only too pleased to welcome a new person into the fold. They've usually been in the same position and are proud of the gym equipment and so want you to share in that feeling. Nowadays most gyms offer an induction session where a qualified instructor will show you how to use the equipment safely, which of course is good for you and good for the gym, too.*

11

On your bike

It's time to dust the cobwebs off that abandoned fitness equipment you have long since forgotten and see how it can clean up your blood pressure.

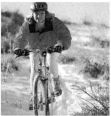

Look in closets, near the back where things are hidden out of sight, or in the attic or the garage. If you can't find anything, you haven't looked hard enough. Try again.

Everyone has some exercise equipment that they have bought or acquired during their life—an exercise ball, dumbbells, an exercise mat, or a jump rope. They looked great on the TV or in the magazine, just like the perfectly toned models who demonstrated how for just $19.99 you could have that perfect *Baywatch* body. So without even getting off your seat, you dialed the toll-free number and started the ball rolling.

Have you found it yet? You have? Good. It's time to dust it off and make it work for you and your blood pressure.

Around six out of ten men, and seven out of ten women, are not active enough to benefit their health. Just 30 minutes of moderately intense physical activity at least

Here's an idea for you...

Once you have found and dusted off the fitness equipment, read the instructions and use it every day. Build up each week by increasing how much you do within the 30 minutes. This will keep you motivated so you will keep enjoying the activity. If you found more than one piece of equipment, use them on alternate weeks.

five days a week reduces the risk of developing diabetes, heart disease, strokes, some cancers, and, of course, high blood pressure. If you already have high blood pressure, then this amount of activity can help you lower it. So no matter what piece of equipment you have, you are going to start using it. You don't have to do 30 minutes at once. You can do smaller blocks, for example, three blocks of 10 minutes—before you go to work, during your lunch break, and when you return home. If this seems too much of a challenge, then do six blocks of 5 minutes to begin with. Just make sure that what you do makes you feel warm and slightly out of breath and that your heart rate increases—you may feel like this sitting watching an aerobics video or DVD but that doesn't count, you have to be physically active at the same time.

I know what you're thinking but you have to resist the urge to go out and buy something new. Before you do that you need to show that you are committed. Remember last Christmas? The "New Year, new you" needed the latest hi-tech rowing machine or exercise bike, so off you went to buy one. You may have even removed it from the box and assembled it. For the first week or two the machine that was to be the answer to all your health and fitness dreams did its best to assist you, but before very long it was just another expensive clothes hanger.

Don't go and buy new equipment for the moment, because you are going to make use of what you already have. After a few months of using the equipment on a regular basis, once you've proven to yourself that you can keep it up, then, and only then, should you consider buying something else. If you've ever joined a gym but a few months later your only contact is paying the membership fee, then you'll understand what I mean. Get into the habit first, make exercise and being active part of your everyday routine, and then consider spending money.

Pedometers are great for motivation. Walk through IDEA 13, *Pedometers*, to find out more.

Try another idea...

You could borrow some fitness equipment from a friend if they are not using it. They will probably be pleased to see it being used—it may help them feel less guilty about having purchased it in the first place. Attention: Do not offer or accept to buy it from them. Not yet anyway. Welcome this abandoned piece of equipment into your life and use it for a total of 30 minutes each day—make sure you know how to use it first so that you do not cause yourself injury.

If you really don't have any fitness equipment then use what you were born with, your legs. Walking, jogging, going up and down stairs, whatever you prefer.

"The most exciting phrase to hear in science, the one that heralds new discoveries, is not 'Eureka!' but 'That's funny...'"
ISAAC ASIMOV

Defining idea...

How did it go?

Q **I got bored of walking the same old route every day. How can I inject some variety?**

A   *Try making it more interesting by walking with a friend or by listening to music as you walk. Change your route each day to keep it interesting. In some areas health educators have created healthy walking guides that offer a good level of activity while introducing people to places of interest at the same time. Try to find out if they are available in your area. Alternatively, vary what activity you do each week, or simply change to another activity for a while and then return to walking later on.*

Q **I couldn't resist, I went out and bought a cross-trainer. Am I an abject failure?**

A   *Not at all! First of all, channel any of the guilt you are feeling into positive energy. Remove your new toy from it's packaging, assemble it, and make sure you put it somewhere where it is visible so that you don't forget that you have it. And never, ever hang clothes on it. Read the instructions carefully and get going. Set a regular time when you intend to use it. If at any stage you start to falter, put something to attract you into the room, a radio or a TV where you can listen to or watch a favorite program. Be careful not to just go through the motions. It's easy when using a cross-trainer, or exercise bike, or rowing machine, for example, to be watching the TV, and although you are moving, you are not putting in enough effort to gain any benefit.*

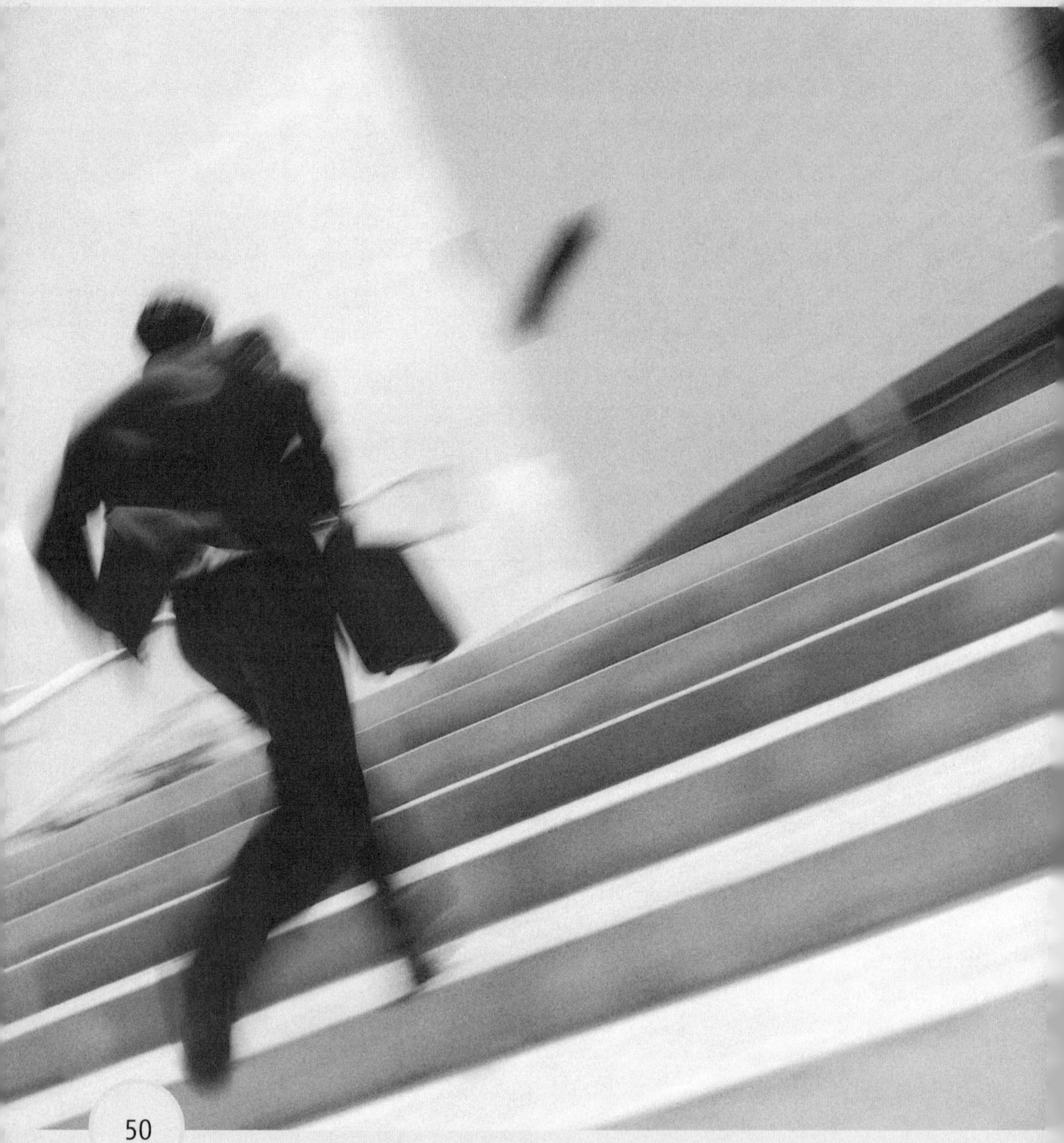

12

Off the bus, up the stairs

Not getting any exercise because you're stuck in front of the computer all day? Did you know it's possible to exercise during the workday without even thinking about it?

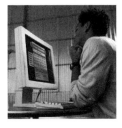

Just take a moment to think about your typical workday. You get up, use the bathroom, hopefully you eat breakfast, get the kids off to school.

You read the morning paper at breakfast or on your way to work. The bus, train, or car transports you, and when you arrive perhaps you get into the elevator. You make coffee in the staff kitchen, and then switch on your computer or whatever equipment you use. OK, so this may not exactly be the start to your workday but it's probably close enough.

Ask people why they don't exercise on workdays and the usual response is that they just don't have the time: We're working longer hours, with greater workloads and tighter deadlines. Now experts recommend doing 30 minutes of moderately intense physical activity on at least five days of the week to help reduce the risk of health problems such as high blood pressure. Like algebra (remember algebra?), at first

Here's an idea for you...

You probably have meetings every now and then at work. You may have them every day. If you are having a meeting, or even just gossiping with one or two other colleagues, rather than sitting around a table or standing still, try walking while you are talking.

glance this time and motion equation doesn't seem to work. But there are solutions.

To begin with, the 30 minutes doesn't have to be all at once. It can be 15-minute, 10-minute, or even 5-minute blocks. It doesn't need to be exercise as such. It's activity that is important. Getting up and going to see a colleague rather than sending an email, going to a local coffee shop to get your midmorning coffee rather than making it in the staff kitchen, these all count toward the 30 minutes of activity. You don't need to be sweating and panting, you just need to feel warm, feel slightly out of breath, and for your heartbeat to increase.

So let's return to your workday routine, because this is the key, making these beneficial activities part of your routine.

At each stage of your day think about how you can change what you are doing so that you are more active doing it. For example, instead of having your morning newspaper delivered, walk to the newsstand and buy it. Perhaps you could walk with your children to school. They'll certainly benefit from this. Could you walk or bike to work? If not, think about getting off the bus one stop earlier and walking the rest of the way. Use the stairs rather than the elevator, or if you don't need the elevator take a slightly longer route to your work area. Each time you have to use the stairs go up and down twice instead of just once. You'll soon feel your heart rate increasing when you do this. Rather than leaning against the photocopier, walk to and from your desk while it's churning out those vital documents. Try taking a slightly longer route to the copier, and walk briskly. These all count. Amazing, isn't it? In fact, by lunchtime you could have already done your 30 minutes.

These are simple ideas, aren't they? It didn't take much effort either. Try IDEA 16, *Remove the remote, mobilize the mobile*, because this is even easier.

Try another idea...

Although many people seem to be able to go all day without using the bathroom, again because they are too busy, the reality is we all need to go during the day. So try this. When you need to use the bathroom, if possible, use one on a different floor from the one you usually use, or use one that is farther away—you may want to practice this during times when you don't need to go so that you don't get caught short. You could also try going to the bathroom every one to two hours, whether you feel the need to go or not. You see, if you walk briskly there and back you could easily be achieving 25 percent of the day's activity requirement doing something you should be doing anyway.

"A man's health can be judged by which he takes two at a time—pills or stairs."
JOAN WELSH

Defining idea...

How did it go?

Q   **We don't have a local coffee shop, and my boss doesn't like employees to leave the building. How can I turn my caffeine fix into an activity?**

A   *OK, but I presume your boss doesn't mind you having a coffee or tea break. Here's what you do. Take a longer route to the kitchen. Ask colleagues if you can make them a cup, but don't phone or email them, actually walk and do the rounds collecting the orders. While the kettle is boiling, jog on the spot or walk briskly around the workplace, maybe walk up and down the stairs. You see, you can be active during time that you would probably have been standing still, time that your boss accepts you need to have away from your workstation. What you are doing is making good use of the time.*

Q   **I'm always running late for work. How can I find the time to do these things in the morning?**

A   *I'm guessing that getting up a little bit earlier to create some time is not possible for you. You can be more active during the day in the ways we've already talked about. Moreover, if it's hard for you to do these things at the beginning of the day, do them at the end of the day. Use the stairs when you leave work, don't get on the bus at your usual stop but walk to the next stop, and also get off one stop earlier. If you drive to work, then park your car farther from your workplace than you normally would.*

13

Pedometers

It's not about how long your workout is, it's about how many steps you're taking. Pedometers are the newest fashion accessory that everyone wants to be seen wearing.

It's said to be almost the perfect exercise. No equipment needed, no expense, and it's there in front of you. Walking, the most ideal exercise in the world, probably.

Yes, walking counts toward the exercise we should all be doing each day. Walking up the stairs, walking to the store and back, even walking around the house. It all counts.

The experts say we should all aim for 10,000 steps a day. Do you have any idea how many steps you take each day? Apparently, on average most of us only make it to a measly three or four thousand a day. Cars, buses, and trains have a lot to answer for. So do computers and phones. We've all become far less active, and physically lazy.

Here's an idea for you... **Write down how many steps you think you take during each day of the week. Then get a pedometer and see how close you were with your estimate and how close you are to the 10,000 steps a day target. If you're already there, congratulations! Now try increasing the target by 500 steps each week. If you're not quite there yet, keep on trying.**

Now you could count how many steps you take throughout the day in your head, but how sad would that be? Do you want to be known in your neighborhood as that weird guy who goes around counting to himself? It's up to you, but there's a much easier way! Here's something for the gadget lovers among you, and even the technophobes out there will come to enjoy the latest strap-on accessory that everyone's wearing.

THESE BOOTS ARE MADE FOR WALKING

Previously confined to specialty stores, pedometers are now available at a store near you. It's not a new idea but with home health monitoring products becoming ever more popular, the simple pedometer is stamping its ground. Blood pressure monitors, home blood testing kits, even a service whereby your heart rate and rhythm can be recorded at home and interpreted by a specialist on the other end of the phone, are in people's homes. Now it's time for the pedometer to come home, too.

So how does this little gadget work? It's simple. The device is the size of a pager and clips onto your belt. It consists of a motion-sensitive electronic circuit. As your body moves, a spring-set horizontal arm turns this electrical circuit on and off, activating the digital counter to clock and record each step taken. Some detect vertical hip movement, others detect the impact of your foot each time it hits the ground.

Older models only measured steps. Newer all-singing, all-dancing models also record the distance walked and the calories burned. Take note, the calorie counting is sometimes over-generous.

Want to get more steps out of your day? Trot along to IDEA 12, *Off the bus, up the stairs*, and find out how you can.

Try another idea...

Pedometers are great motivators. They provide instant, effortless feedback on how well you've done. You'll want to hit that 10,000 target each day, and then you'll want to score even more. If you find it hard to spend 30 minutes each day being physically active, even if you can't manage three blocks of 10 minutes, then a pedometer may be just the thing for you.

How fancy the pedometer you choose is depends on what you want from it and the type of person you are. If you're a gadget freak, then I'm sure you'll want a pedometer that does everything and more. Many pedometers have a stopwatch function, an alarm function, can even talk…if only they could pour you a drink when you come home! But they won't do the walking for you, and you'll need to pony up a little more cash for these hi-tech versions. Likewise if you're serious about knowing how far you walk and want a reliable calories-burned figure, it'll cost you more. Be honest with yourself—if you have trouble programming your TiVO, then stick with a basic pedometer. It'll give you an accurate figure of how many steps you've taken, which is, after all, what you want from it.

"The sovereign invigorator of the body is exercise, and of all the exercises walking is the best."
THOMAS JEFFERSON

Defining idea...

How did it go?

Q **I'm nowhere near 10,000 a day. Got any simple ideas on how I can step up?**

A *Each day aim to increase the number of steps you take by just 100. Walk up and down the stairs twice instead of once, take a slightly longer route to the store or to the printer in the office. Rather than sending memos to your work colleagues by email, deliver them personally. After a month of doing this you will have increased your walking by 3,000 steps, after two months by 6,000 steps, and so on. Before very long you will be easily clocking 10,000 steps a day and starting to achieve even more.*

Q **My pedometer keeps falling off. Any tips for preventing this?**

A *If there's one thing that's likely to make you want to throw your pedometer in the trash, it's the fact that it keeps falling off. Some pedometers have a nasty habit of doing this around toilets. Wearing a thinner or thicker belt may help the clip fit more securely. Try putting a safety string through the pedometer clip and attach this to your belt or clothing. This way at least if the pedometer slips off the belt you won't lose it.*

Q **Where can I get a pedometer?**

A *Sports equipment stores usually have a good range of pedometers to choose from. Some pharmacies, department stores, and electronics stores are now stocking them, too. Since pedometers are becoming more popular many companies, e.g., cereal and food manufacturers, are offering them to their customers.*

14

Weekend wonders

Things to do, places to be, people to see. Of course the weekend is good for you, but if you play your cards right it can be good for your blood pressure, too.

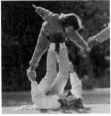

The weekend is the time when you're allowed to relax and unwind. The word spells it out, and tells you that the working week is now at an end.

It's when you are supposed to take time out for yourself, to recharge your batteries for the next week.

It's during the weekend that many of us actually achieve the recommended 30 minutes of moderately intensive physical activity a day. Ironic really, isn't it? The time when we are supposed to be resting is the time when we are probably most physically active.

This shouldn't come as a surprise though. Chores that would have been done sometime during the week have now been pushed onto the weekend. You are too busy to cut the lawn, do the shopping, do the laundry, and tidy the house during the week. So these become weekend fixtures. Of course, that's along with visiting

Here's an idea for you... **Try not using the car on weekends. Walk to the park or to visit friends instead. If it's too far, drive part of the way and then walk the rest. It may seem inconvenient at first, especially if your weekend is spent taking the children here, there, and everywhere, but doing this will benefit you and the kids, too.**

friends and taking the children to parties, dance lessons, and sports events. Oh, and having a night out. One way or another it all gets packed in.

You could say that this isn't good. Well, it isn't if come Monday morning you're exhausted and feeling like it's Friday already. However, take heart: You may be doing just what the doctor ordered, or to be medico-politically correct, what the doctor advised. Cutting the lawn, digging the garden, painting your fence all count as healthy activity. If the weekend is when you enjoy a round of golf—particularly if you pull or carry your own bag—a game of badminton, or a swim at the local pool, then keep it up.

But what if you are a weekend couch potato? Your weekend consists of staying in bed—but no sex. A pity because a portion, or all, of the recommended 30 minutes activity could be achieved before you even get out of bed. What a wonderful prescription! Once you are up and out of bed a leisurely breakfast with the Saturday paper is followed by the rest of the day on the phone to friends or watching the sports channel on TV. OK, so you do leave your home in the evening to go out to the bar but the only activity there is going to and from the bar. Well, that would be a start, but you are hardly going to be walking briskly and these days table service eliminates the need for you to even stand...not that you are likely to be able to do this as the evening progresses.

Well, here's something for you couch potatoes to try. What you do during the day isn't really going to change, so don't panic. It's how you do it that needs to change. Start off by going to the newsstand to buy your Saturday paper rather than having it delivered. Walk to the store, don't use the car. If you already do this, take a longer route there and back and walk briskly, or even jog. When on the phone, walk around while you're talking. Better still, walk outside in the yard so you have more space. Don't use the remote: Get up to change TV channels. Did you know that a four-hour retail therapy outing to get something for your night out will notch up around 10,000 steps—your target for the day. What more could you want!? In the evening, why not walk to the bar, club, bingo, or wherever you choose to while away your time. You spend a lot of time thinking about where to go and what to wear, so choose somewhere where you can dance: This is a great activity. By getting into the routine of being more active in this way you won't even have to think about it.

Everybody's working for the weekend, so let's see how to make taking care of your blood pressure pure pleasure. It's time for you to enjoy IDEA 9, *Active hedonism*.

Try another idea...

"People rarely succeed unless they have fun in what they are doing."
DALE CARNEGIE

Defining idea...

61

Q **I work a six-day week. It's difficult for me to do very much on my one day off. How can I fit in some activity?**

A *Try putting the ideas discussed above into practice on your working days. Remember, the target is to be moderately physically active for 30 minutes on at least five days of the week. You don't have to achieve it every day, although of course this would be good.*

Q **I'm using the supermarket for one-stop weekly shopping so I'm less active, I know. Any ideas?**

A *Try doing some or all of your shopping at speciality stores and farmers' markets. If you continue using the supermarket one alternative is to use a pushcart and walk part or all of the way there and back. Another good idea is to simply park your car at the far side of the supermarket parking lot rather than as close as you can get to the entrance.*

Q **I spend a lot of time gardening and doing home-improvement projects on weekends. Is this enough?**

A *Well done! If you want to be a little more active try putting electrical tools and equipment to one side and doing the work using traditional ones. Use shears rather than your electric hedge trimmer, a brush rather than a vacuum, and a handsaw rather than an electric one, for example.*

15

Do the shake and vac

Housework doesn't have to be a chore. Really, it doesn't. Making it work for you can put the freshness back into your blood pressure.

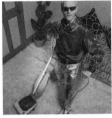

Ironing. You either love it or you loathe it. If there's one domestic activity that can help cement a relationship it's having one partner who is happy to iron clothes.

Even with modern-day fabric technology that teases us with "easy-iron" labels, or even "no ironing needed," the reality is that in a world where we like to wear a freshly pressed item of clothing, ironing is here to stay.

Are you ready for this? It's time for some good news to come out of all that heat and steam. Ironing counts as a valuable activity with regards to blood pressure and general health. And so do many other daily activities that you do without thinking about it. Yes, you read that correctly, your glasses have not steamed up. So should you be gathering up every piece of clothing you can find, advertising in the local paper for ironing jobs, even ironing underwear? Well, you can if you want, but it's not necessary.

Here's an idea for you... **Be more active around the house. If you're downstairs use the bathroom upstairs, and vice versa. Move up the stairs briskly. Get up to answer the phone and walk around while talking. Open the door yourself rather than buzzing the person in. You'll be surprised how easy it is to do these simple but effective activities.**

In the quest to achieve 30 minutes of moderately intense physical activity on at least five days a week, activity that will not only help keep blood pressure at a safe level, but that will also make you feel good, housework—among other indoor activities—counts. So housework should be something to embrace and look forward to. Well, maybe not. But you may find it easier if you look upon it as being good for you rather than a chore. After all, these things have to be done, so you might as well get the best out of them.

Take ironing for example. Please, take my ironing, I hear you cry. Picture this. You are sitting with a pile of ironing in front of the TV gently passing the iron back and forth across the clothes. You may already be standing and rhythmically your arm is flowing from side to side. Instead of watching TV while ironing, listen to music and put a bit more effort into it. You'll find yourself being a little more energetic. You may even start, dare I say it, enjoying it. Heaven forbid!

Of course, this only counts as light exercise, but it's a start. Dusting and cleaning count as light exercise, too, but it depends on how energetic you are. Cleaning windows, for example, is more active, but best of all is vacuuming, which counts as a moderately intense activity. Dance around while you are doing it and you'll really be contributing to your 30 minutes. And that goes for men, too—but make sure you put some effort into it. Don't spend most of the time pretending to be a rock star.

Many people now work from home. This has its good and bad points. One of the benefits of working from home is that sometimes it's easier to get everyday things done; the laundry for example. However, it's also easy for you to be spending hours sitting in front of the computer or on the phone. I know someone who decided to see how well he was doing with regards to achieving his target 10,000 steps a day. He was shocked to find that in the course of one day at home he barely achieved 500 steps, a long way from the target. One thing he did to improve this was to simply go up and down stairs regularly throughout the day. It provided him with a natural break from the computer screen, meant that he drank more liquid during the day, and he found to his surprise that he worked more efficiently.

OK, it's time to take a short break. Have a look at IDEA 39, *Pet project*, to see how pets can help you make the best of this time.

Try another idea...

"Though no one can go back and make a brand-new start, anyone can start from now and make a brand-new ending."
CARL BARD

Defining idea...

How did it go?

Q **I'm not really very good at cooking and don't have the time to cook when I get in from work. What's wrong with living on takeout?**

A *Living on takeout may be convenient but isn't particularly good for your blood pressure since many of the foods have a high salt content. They are also usually high in fat, too, so are not good for your blood vessels. One thing you could do to help your blood pressure, until your culinary circumstances change, is to go and pick up the meal yourself rather than have it delivered—and walk to the restaurant, don't drive!*

Q **I have a cleaner so I don't do the housework thing. What can I do? I don't want to fire my cleaner.**

A *If, like many people, you clean and tidy up before your cleaner comes, you may already be quite active on the housework front. If you let your cleaner do all the work, then presumably this is to save you time, so why not find a hobby or another pleasurable activity that you can spend this time on?*

Q **I seem to spend most of my time in the kitchen. How can I be more active?**

A *Try not using all those culinary gadgets! For example, when baking, instead of placing the ingredients into the food processor, beat the mixture yourself using a wooden spoon. And keep moving, too. It's estimated than one hour's cooking in the kitchen involves taking around 3,000 steps, almost a third of the daily 10,000-step target.*

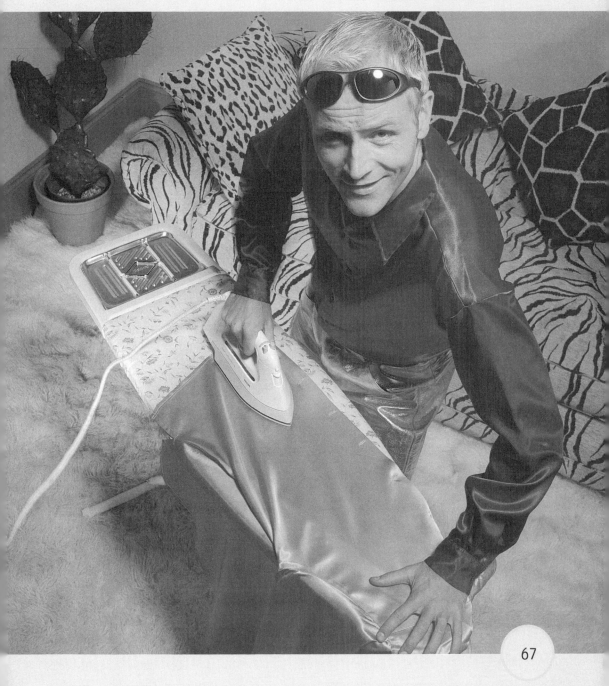

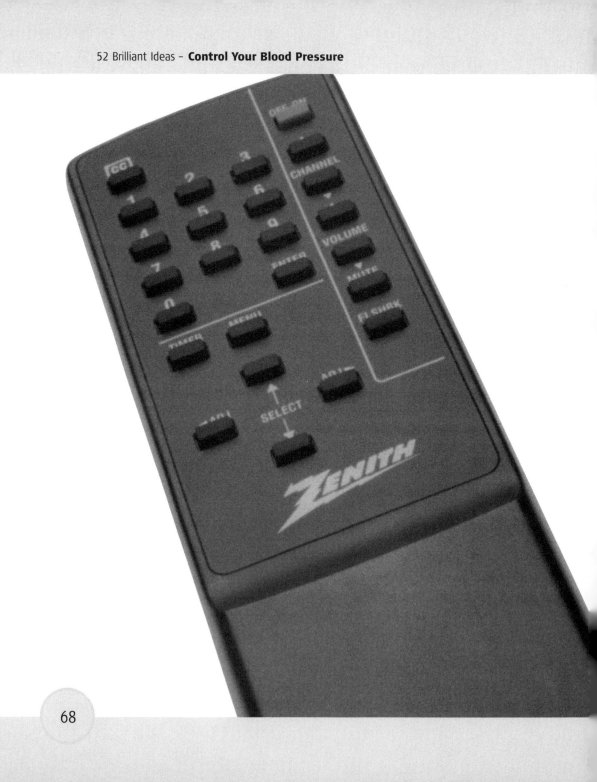

16

Remove the remote, mobilize the mobile

Where's the remote? The cry heard from living rooms everywhere. Don't get frustrated though, because getting off your backside is good for you and your blood pressure.

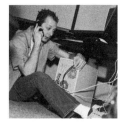

So the remote is no longer by your side where it should be? This means your television viewing is going to be disturbed, and so is your position of relaxed tranquility.

Yep, whether the remote is just out of reach or lost, you are going to have to lift yourself off the couch.

There's scientific evidence to suggest that just by getting up from the couch to change channels or alter the volume on a regular basis, you can lower your blood pressure. Although it may not seem like much, you are increasing your activity levels by doing something that wouldn't ordinarily happen if the remote was planted on your sofa. So you can see why it's actually better for the remote to be temporarily, or indeed permanently, lost. OK, I agree that it's stressful when you can't get your hands on the remote, and this in itself may temporarily increase

Here's an idea for you... **Put the remote out of reach. Somewhere where it's quicker for you to get up and manually change channels. Soon doing this will become a habit, you'll be changing channels like in the old days, and helping your blood pressure into the bargain.**

blood pressure and potentially counteract the benefits of being up and about, but take a deep breath and you'll be winning all the way.

After the arrival of the remote control there was a brief time when technology gave us a break. For a while remote controls were not all bad news. One remote for the television, one for the VCR, one for the DVD, another for the satellite system…there was always one that you'd have to get up to find! The more you have, the more you have to lose, right? But the arrival of multifunctional remotes means you can now close the curtains, feed the cat, and mow the lawn from the touchscreen comfort of that buttock-shaped depression in your sofa.

Whatever did people do before remote controls? Kept fit, that's what! No remote meant no stress for you about not having it. Having to get up and down meant your weight would have been a little less. Those around you would have been happier since you would have been less likely to be driving them crazy with your channel surfing. And if you had managed to channel surf without a remote, then that in itself would have been impressive feat and a decent amount of exercise.

Modern communications need to shoulder some of the blame for high blood pressure, obesity, and a general decline in physical fitness, too. Remember those days when if the phone rang you'd have to go to it? Think a little further back and you may recall having to go outside to a pay phone when you wanted to make a call. The arrival of cordless and mobile phones has meant that such activities are no longer necessary. Like our good friend the remote control, the phone can always be by our side so the most we have to do is a single finger press and raise an arm.

All this getting up and down has got you moving. Look at IDEA 15, *Do the shake and vac,* to see where else in the house you can get active.

Try another idea...

But don't hang the phones up yet; think about this idea. Keep your cordless phone in its base unit rather than beside you within easy reach. Keep your mobile phone away from you, too. If you work in an office, put the cell somewhere away from your own desk. The principle behind this is that, as with the remote control, you have to move to answer the call. In addition, while talking on the phone, try walking around. A phone call that lasts twenty minutes will clock up around 2,000 steps. That's a fifth of the recommended daily walk. You'd be on the phone anyway, so it's not as though it's going to interfere with what you are doing. You're benefitting your blood pressure for minimal effort—could it be easier?

"The human body has been designed to resist an infinite number of changes and attacks brought about by its environment. The secret of good health lies in successful adjustment to changing stresses on the body."
HARRY J. JOHNSON

Defining idea...

How did it go?

Q   I work in an open-plan office and if I leave my cell phone away from my desk, my colleagues complain that it's disturbing them. When it rings they think it's theirs! What can I do?

A   *This is why God created a range of ringtones! Find a distinctive but non-irritating one. Otherwise, you'll just have to keep your cell with you, but get up and walk around your desk once before answering it. You could put it on the floor on the far side of your desk so that you still have to get up to answer it.*

Q   My desk phone is on a landline and isn't cordless. What can I do?

A   *Stand up to answer the phone and walk in place. Alternatively, get an extension telephone cord so you can walk around while you talk. Nowadays we spend so much time on the phone it's a shame not to take advantage of this opportunity. Think about it, ten 10-minute phone calls could clock up your day's activity quota.*

Q   I hid the remote and my family was furious. How can I restore calm?

A   *Obviously this wasn't the best time to try this idea, as others in your household were clearly not ready to take this courageous step with you. You could encourage them to follow suit though. Tell them how it will help you and them.*

17

Get the gear

You're ready for action so you need to look good. Now it's time to buy the gear. If you want to get the best and not end up bankrupt, read on.

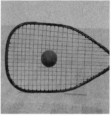

The right gear and the right equipment are essential. You need to look like a professional with the right branding, and this season's colors. Of course.

But just take a time-out to think about why are you becoming more active. It's because you want your blood pressure to be at a safe level. So in addition to making you look good, what you wear and the equipment you use must look after you. It's easy to buy the training shoes that are the most fashionable, but what's most important is that they fit correctly and feel comfortable. You don't want your activity to be cut short by blisters and injuries. Likewise, clothing should be comfortable, too. There's a huge psychological and motivational boost to wearing sports clothing that you feel good in. Likewise, there's not much chance of you being enthusiastic if you would feel more comfortable in sackcloth.

Before blowing your month's salary on everything you see that's related to your chosen activity, check out some books or a few websites to see what is the

Here's an idea for you... **Visit as many sports shops as you can before purchasing anything. This will allow you to actually find out what's available and how good it feels and looks on you. Remember, it has to feel comfortable and look fantastic. Walking around the different stores is also valuable activity. A 4-hour shopping trip equates to around 10,000 steps, your target for a day.**

minimum you need. According to writer Erma Bombeck, "The odds of going to the store for a loaf of bread and coming out with *only* a loaf of bread are three billion to one." So when the salesman is trying to sell you everything from a portable refrigerator to an inflatable stretcher, ask him to prioritize the list in order of importance, or better still, ask him what the minimum is that you need to get started.

Don't feel rushed either. Yes, I know you don't want to lose your momentum, but you want to enjoy the experience, too. Trying on the different sportswear, handling the equipment—it should be like enjoying a fine wine. Take your time. Savor the moment. You want to get it right. This is why a little research is helpful. If you are going to be playing a club-based sport—tennis, for example—ask the other players what they recommend. Sometimes they will have equipment available for you to try or even to purchase used.

Nowadays it's easy to sit in front of the computer and get good deals. But before you go click, click, click, and wait expectantly for the mail, again do your research. If the Internet offers the best deal, then go for it. Just make sure that a few mouse clicks isn't all the activity you do.

After all that shopping you'll be needing a pick-me-up. Have a sip of IDEA 31, *Hey there, smoothie.*

Try another idea...

A common problem in sporting activities is the false start. It may be that after trying an activity for a while, despite thinking it was right for you, it clearly isn't. Perhaps circumstances have gotten in the way and despite wanting to take part it just isn't possible. To add insult to injury—and injury may be exactly why you can't be involved—you now have a bag full of costly clothing and equipment sitting idly like a rebellious teenager, snickering at you every time you look at it. There is a way of avoiding this. Before actually splurging, try to borrow the gear from a friend. This way you will be able to actually try out the equipment and give it a test run. Should you decide to buy your own, don't buy the most expensive to begin with. Again, this way if you should stop using it you're less likely to feel that you have wasted your money. Moreover, you can use thirst for new gear as a motivating factor. Why not decide that once you have been involved in the activity for, let's say, six months, you can upgrade your equipment? This way you always have another goal, in addition to having a good blood pressure reading and being healthy, to spur you on.

"You win some, you lose some, and some get rained out, but you gotta suit up for them all."
J. ASKENBERG

Defining idea...

75

How did it go?

Q **I find it difficult not to buy everything at once. What can I do?**

A *It's easy to get caught up in the flow and spend, spend, spend. Consequently you end up getting as much exercise carrying your bag of equipment to and from the gym, court, or wherever, as you do actually taking part—that is if you have any energy left to take part once you arrive. Make a list of the equipment you think that you need and check off the things you really can't do without. So basically you are prioritizing. Anything that remains unchecked is unnecessary and should be left in the store.*

Q **Tried prioritizing. Failed! How can I curb my uncontrollable urge to buy more equipment?**

A *It sounds as though once you have bought another sport shirt, or bag, or pair of wristbands you still don't feel satisfied. In fact, you probably feel guilty that you should spend more time actually taking part in the activity and less time shopping for equipment. It's OK to buy equipment so long as you can afford it, so long as you need it, and so long as you deserve it. Try setting yourself a target for each week, or each month, whichever you prefer. Once you have played the sport, or been to the gym, or completed 10,000 steps, on at least five days a week for a month, then give yourself permission to buy something.*

18

Body mass index

You've heard it bandied around and you're sure it's not a new rock band. I am a 24. But do you know your number, and what it means?

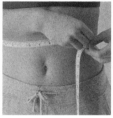

Life is full of numbers. House numbers, phone numbers, lottery numbers. Here's one that's important: your BMI. Introduce yourself, knowing it may save your life.

There's a new kid on the block and he wants to be part of your group. This new kid is basically OK, so long as you keep an eye on him. If you are not careful, though, he's likely to become a little too big for his boots. You see, he fancies himself as a leader, he wants to weigh you down and to take control from you. If you let this happen he'll slowly eat away at your authority, and if his progress is not halted, he'll be your downfall. You may have met this new kid already. He goes by the name of BMI.

It's hard to avoid references to obesity these days. They're everywhere. News programs remind us about how more and more of the population are now classified as overweight or obese. Like the TV preachers who will save our soul for just $9.99, ads and diet programs promise that for a small contribution to the cause they will

Here's an idea for you...

Making sure the curtains are closed, get naked. Weigh yourself (W) and multiply it by 703. Measure your height (H). Divide your weight equation (W) by your height (H). Voilà, the result is your BMI. You can do this in your head or use an online BMI calculator.

show us the way to losing weight and to a healthier, happier you.

Inflation will steadily increase if it's not managed properly, and so will weight. It's a simple equation. *For weight to remain the same "calories in" must equal "calories out."* Food provides the "calories in" part of the equation; exercise or activity provides the "calories out." More in and less out means the equation tips toward increasing weight. Less in and more out means your weight decreases. Currently, for more and more people the balance of this equation is toward too many calories and not enough exercise. Consequently, weight increases. In fact, you don't need to do equations to learn this. Just take a look around you. Seats on buses and trains for two people no longer seem big enough for more than one. Go into a coffee shop and it's not just people's coattails that are hanging over the side of the chair they are sitting on; their buttocks are, too.

We all have a BMI, or body mass index to give it its full name. You may already know yours. Doctors have been making reference to it for years. Insurance and loan companies and the like are now asking for it. Who knows, in the future transport companies may use BMI to rate seat prices.

Being overweight puts you at risk of many health problems. You know that. Blood pressure, for example, is more likely to go up under the pressure of weight. It's harder for the heart to do its job if it has to cope with the additional load of excess weight. The BMI is just a figure that gives an indication of whether you are overweight or not, and if so how much risk being overweight is for your health.

This may have come as a bit of a shock so have a look at IDEA 6, *Chill*, to see how to make the living easy.

Try another idea…

A BMI of 25 or more means you are overweight, a BMI over 30 means that you are clinically obese. The higher the BMI, the greater the risk of health problems.

Reading this your heart is beating a little faster than usual, perhaps there's a bead of sweat on your brow. OK, it's time. You're going to find out what your BMI is. Remember, before you do, if it's higher than it should be there are lots of chapters in this book you should read that will help you to bring your BMI down. Even if you don't yet know your exact BMI figure, a look in the mirror will give you a good idea of whether it's high or not.

"Today is your day, your mountain is waiting, so get on your way."
DR. SEUSS

Defining idea…

How did it go?

Q   What is a normal BMI?

A   *Any reading between 18.5 and 24.9 is considered a safe and healthy BMI. Below 18.5 is underweight, and 25 and above is overweight. Check your BMI each month and, over time, by changing to a healthier lifestyle you should see your BMI either remain in the safety zone, or drop down into this zone.*

Q   Does having a high BMI always mean problems are heading your way?

A   *No, not always. It is possible for two people to have the same BMI and for one to be more at risk of developing health problems than the other. For example, since BMI is calculated using only height and weight it is possible for a fit and muscular person, for example, to have the same BMI and be less at risk of problems than someone with the same BMI but higher body fat levels.*

Q   How important is BMI?

A   *Your BMI serves as a guide but it is only one part of your health profile. It's a good guide, since as BMI increases so does the risk of developing many diseases, such as type 2 diabetes, heart disease, and some cancers. If someone has other risk factors, then their risk will be even greater. The BMI is something that is simple to calculate and to monitor and as such makes it easy for you monitor how well you are doing with achieving your ideal weight.*

19

The fat of the land

Body fat is bad. At least, that's most people's perception. But body fat is not all bad. Let's get a feel for why some body fat can be good.

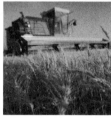

Mention the word "fat" and people shudder, thinking diets must be no fat, bodies must be fat-free, and that fat is an evil being that must be avoided at all cost.

Years ago fat was a treat, something to be enjoyed, eaten with bread. Now the pendulum has swung the other way. Too far the other way because fats are not all bad. In fact, the body needs some fat from food. Fat is necessary for energy reserves. It provides vitamins such as A, D, and E, and essential fatty acids.

There's a lot of talk about body fat percentage. This is the amount of fat tissue in your body as a percentage of total body weight. If the scales say you weigh 200 pounds and you have 40 pounds of fat, your body fat percentage is 20 percent.

This fat, which lies under the skin and surrounds the body, and is often found in more places than in others, has many different functions. It's necessary for body protection—it's our own personal cushion against the world. It insulates the organs

Here's an idea for you...

Figure out your body fat percentage. A quick way is to use a body fat scale or bioelectrical impedance analyzer. These are appearing in pharmacies and gyms, and can also be purchased for home use. Tracking your body fat is the best way to make sure that you're losing fat and gaining muscle. Just don't test it too often, since body fat measurements don't show small changes. Every 4–8 weeks is best.

and tissues of the body and is involved in temperature regulation. In some cultures fat represents success and wealth. In other cultures it makes us cuddly and loveable, giving us something to hold on to.

Those love handles may make us smile but they also represent an indication of potential future illness. The higher your percentage of fat above average levels, the higher your risk of weight-related illness such as osteoarthritis, type 2 diabetes, and high blood pressure.

Your body fat percentage is also important with regards to losing weight. You may have really made an effort to lose some weight by eating sensibly and getting lots of exercise only to find that your weight doesn't fall. In fact, it may have even increased. It's possible that you have been losing fat, which is actually what we want to happen when we say we are trying to lose weight, but have been building muscle mass (which is heavier). Athletes may be overweight but not over-fat. The converse of this is you may have been fooling yourself when you say that your increase in weight is muscle, not fat.

So how can you find out just what your percentage of body fat is? Scales, callipers, or a simple look in the mirror is often enough. The most accurate methods involve high-tech equipment, which usually isn't available outside of a medical or research setting. Dual energy X-ray absorptiometry or DEXA, the method used to measure bone mineral density, can be used to measure fat percentage, and also to determine where most of your fat is—as if this is something you don't already know. DEXA uses a whole body scanner and two different low-dose X-rays to read bone mass and soft tissue mass.

So maybe you're cuddly but have a little fat to lose. Try IDEA 32, *Drop some pounds*, to find out how.

Try another idea...

Another method is hydrostatic weighing, or drowning on scales as it might perhaps be called. Yes, you're right. In this one you get wet. You sit on a scale inside a tank of water and blow out as much air as you can. Next you are dunked under the water and blow out more air. (At this point, try to banish thoughts of Norwegians bearing harpoons.) Fat is lighter than water so the more you have the more you will float.

Skin fold thickness can be measured with callipers. Measurements are usually taken from four places around the body—triceps, biceps, under the shoulder blade, and just above the hip—you know, where you might try to "pinch an inch." The measurements are put into a formula to calculate your body fat. Not as accurate as DEXA or hydrostatic weighing, but more accessible.

"It's simple; if it jiggles, it's fat."
ARNOLD SCHWARZENEGGER

Defining idea...

How did it go?

Q   Do I have to measure my body fat?

A   Measuring body fat percentage isn't necessary for most people. Calculating your body mass index (BMI) or measuring your waist is usually quite sufficient. However, if you wish to measure your body fat, a professional body fat monitor or a scale with a built-in body fat calculator should do the trick.

Q   What is a normal body fat percentage?

A   There's no clear consensus on what is a healthy body fat percentage. Generally speaking, for men, an average is 10–18 percent of body weight, for women it's 18–25 percent. Just as too little body fat can create some pretty devastating physiological complications, too much body fat can have equally harmful effects. Once men creep up over 25 percent and women over 31 percent fat, there is a dramatic correlation with illness and disease.

Q   How do body fat analyzers work?

A   Some are handheld, others look like a bathroom scale that you stand on. The faster the signal passes from hand to hand or from foot to foot, the more muscle you have. The results are based on the fact that water conducts electricity. Fat contains almost no water while muscle is about 70 percent water. Be sure you test at the same time of day, preferably first thing in the morning before breakfast, but after a glass of water. If you're dehydrated, your body fat percentage will read higher than it is.

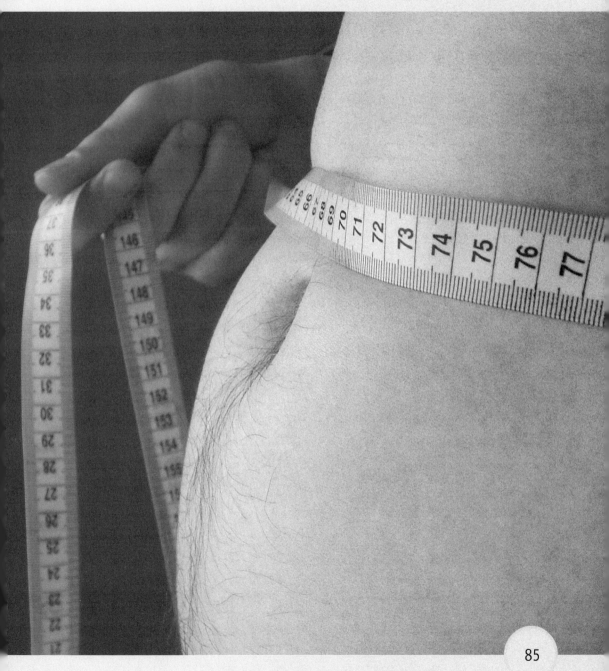

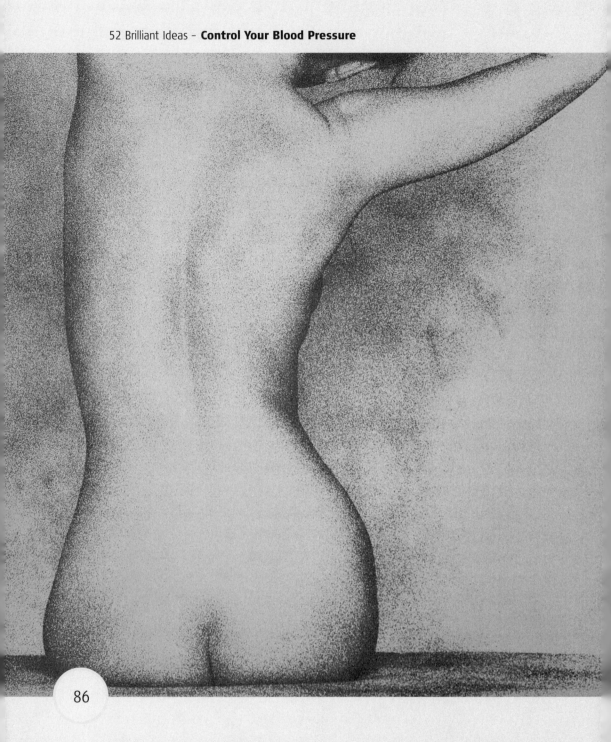

20

Apples and pears

We all know fruit is good for us. But the current buzz is not about vitamin content but about shape. How good is it for your blood pressure if you look like an apple or a pear?

"Oranges and lemons say the bells of St. Clements." This is a line from a well-known nursery rhyme. It's still sung today in playgrounds everywhere.

Many believe the rhyme describes poverty in London, others believe it's about sex. Whatever the meaning, it's time for these fruits to take a bow and move over. Today it's apples and pears that are being proclaimed the new stars of the show.

Apples and pears are great to eat, and eating an average-size portion of each a day can make up around 40 percent of the recommended daily five portions of fruits and vegetables. So far, so good. Here's the catch though: The new rise to fame for these fruits is not their content or the fact that they are good for us. No. It's their shape, or to put it bluntly, how similar our body shape is to theirs, and how that can be bad news.

Here's an idea for you...

Following the instructions, calculate your waist–hip ratio. Soon you'll know whether you're an apple or a pear, and whether you need peeling or not. You need to know since this way you can be better prepared and hopefully out of the way when, as the nursery rhyme says, "Here comes the chopper to chop off your head."

Most people store their body fat in two distinct ways. If it's around your middle, that's called apple-shaped; if it's around your hips and thighs, that's called pear-shaped. The shape of your body is directly linked to your risk of bad health. Many scientific studies have identified that carrying extra weight around the stomach brings more risk for your health than carrying extra weight around your hips or thighs. The bottom line: Excess fat in the abdominal region puts you at a greater risk of developing high blood pressure than excess fat in the hips and thighs.

A simple way of assessing your risk is just to look in the mirror. If you have more weight around your waist than around your hips and thighs, that is, your outline is more an apple than a pear, then you have a greater risk of lifestyle-related diseases such as heart disease and diabetes.

Another more technical, but still simple and useful, measure of fat distribution around the body is called the waist-to-hip ratio (WHR). This looks at the proportion of fat stored on your body around your waist and hips.

The best way to do this is while you're standing, relaxed and naked. Measure your waist at its narrowest point. This is usually around your navel. Next, measure your hips at their widest point. This is usually around the buttocks. It's important not to pull the tape tight when doing either of these measurements; let the tape rest on your skin. And here's a special note for men: The waist measurement is made around the level of your belly button, not where your waistband or belt sits, as this may be hiding far below your belly. Finally, divide your waist measurement by your hip measurement.

Since you're in the mood to measure parts of your anatomy try out IDEA 2, *Playing doctors and nurses.*

Try another idea...

The figure you get from this calculation is your WHR. For men, a WHR of more than 1.0 means they are apples. For women the crucial figure is 0.8. More importantly, apples are at greater risk of suffering health-related problems because of this fat distribution.

Being shaped like an apple is also known as having central obesity, or to put it simply, it's what your mother called carrying a bit of a tummy, or your friends call a beer belly. Nowadays, no one wants to have a fat tummy, do they? No, of course they don't. If you are a woman you want a nice flat stomach, if you are a man you probably want a six-pack abdomen. The media promotes this as being desirable. Just look how happy and fit the people with these features are. Happy, smiling faces, in perfect health, with the world, not their belly, at their feet. You want a good-looking tummy for the reason that it makes you feel good about yourself, and that hopefully others will find you attractive, too. But there's a more important reason for having a well-shaped tummy: It may keep you alive longer.

"There are no shortcuts in evolution."
LOUIS D. BRANDEIS, Supreme Court Justice

Defining idea...

89

How did it go?

Q   Is a waist measurement alone helpful?

A   *Yes, it can be since waist circumference on its own also provides a helpful guide to predicting the risk of developing health-related problems such as heart disease. For men, a waist circumference less than 37 inches is OK. Having a waist circumference of 37–39 inches increases the risk of health problems, and of 40 inches or more substantially increases the risk. For Asian men, 36 inches or more substantially increases the risk of health problems. For women, a waist circumference less than 32 inches is OK. Having a waist circumference of 32–34 inches increases the risk of health problems, and of 35 inches or more substantially increases the risk. For Asian females, 32 inches or more substantially increases the risk of health problems.*

Q   Which is more important, not carrying excess weight or having a good waist-to-hip ratio?

A   *Not carrying excess weight is more important with regards to the risk of high blood pressure and, more importantly, of developing heart disease. Overall, obesity puts you at greater risk than where fat is distributed or stored on your body. So long as you avoid excess weight, being an apple not a pear doesn't put you at special risk, but it's something to keep in mind. Even if you are a pear, then you should still make sure that you maintain your ideal weight so you avoid the health problems associated with obesity.*

21

Come on, it's time for breakfast

If you miss breakfast you're missing out big-time. So here's how to make sure you don't miss out on the most important meal of the day.

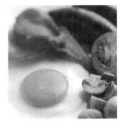

Overnight the body undergoes a mini-fast, around eight to ten hours without food. In the morning by eating we break this fast, hence the name, "breakfast."

That's why when you get up in the morning if you're not feeling hungry right away, you'll certainly want to eat something within an hour or two.

No matter who you are or where you are, your natural instinct is to eat soon after you get up. Eating breakfast not only fulfills this need and is an excellent way to start the day, but getting some healthy food into you first thing will lessen the chance of you suffering the unhealthy snack attacks that assist in raising blood pressure.

Here's an idea for you...

You can do this at home or at work. You *do* have time. Fill the pot to make your first cup of coffee or tea of the day. Now, while the water is boiling prepare and eat a bowl of cereal. You don't have to rush it, take your time and enjoy it.

You know the routine. Jump out of bed, use the bathroom, quick shower, throw on some clothes, and hope that items of clothing that should be in pairs haven't decided to mix and un-match. Grab the keys and out the door.

Meanwhile your stomach is empty. It's feeling hungry and starting to let you know this by sending out familiar hunger sensations. Your brain is not too happy either. Your blood sugar levels will be registering at the lower end of normal, and consequently despite only being out of bed for less than a couple of hours you're already starting to feel tired.

So what do you do? You reach for the nearest snack. Yes, that cake, cookie, or chocolate bar sure does taste good. *Mmmmm.* And it's true that, like a flash, you're feeling back on track. These snacks, although tasty, provide too much sugar, too quickly, leaving you feeling shaky and lethargic rather than supercharged. Before long you'll be reaching for another snack as you ride the sugar roller coaster.

If you don't usually have breakfast, try it. A glass of orange juice, some fruit, a couple of slices of toast, a bowl of cereal are just some of the simple ways to give you a heads-up. They'll give you the sugar boost to get you going, plus they'll give you sugar energy that's released gradually, too, so that you don't start to flag early on. You'll feel better, you'll have more energy, and you'll not be eating so many unhealthy snacks. It's not as difficult as you think. If you only have a banana and a glass of fruit juice, then you've also had two of your target five portions of fruits and vegetables for the day.

Although it's not ideal you could eat something on your way to work. This way you can still stay in bed until that penultimate moment when any longer and you'll be late for work. A few dried apricots, a banana, or a yogurt drink are easy to have on the go. Of course, you could always have breakfast at work. I know many people who have cereal in their desk drawer for this reason. Many places of work have a small kitchen area where toast can be made and food and drinks kept refrigerated. Be honest; will spending ten minutes to have breakfast before you start work make that much difference? In fact, it will mean you are more productive during the rest of the morning so that you'll probably end up saving that time and more.

Most people say they don't have breakfast because they don't have time. This is a poor excuse. You could probably eat a bowl of cereal in the time it took your coffee to brew. You could have eaten a bowl of cereal while your computer booted up, too. This isn't a race against time. Sit and enjoy some breakfast. More importantly, eating breakfast means you won't get those hunger pangs or feel fatigued before your day's work has even begun.

So now you know you have a few minutes available, you might like some more ways to spend these. Try IDEA 38, *Can I have 5 minutes of your time?*

Try another idea...

"It is well to be up before daybreak, for such habits contribute to health, wealth, and wisdom."
ARISTOTLE

Defining idea...

Q I like to have breakfast at the local diner with my friends. We all meet there before starting work. A fully cooked breakfast first thing in the morning is a tradition, isn't it?

A   *At least you're having breakfast. It's OK to have a greasy fried breakfast every now and then, but not every day since it tends to be high in fat and puts weight on you. Asking for grilled rather than fried is a good start. Try whole grain toast, oatmeal, or a poached egg instead. It doesn't have to be a case of when in Rome. Your friends may tease you for opting for a healthier choice, but who knows, they may have been waiting for someone to take the lead, and be grateful to you for getting the ball rolling.*

Q Do you have any idea how long it takes me to get the kids fed and off to school?

A   *You're not going to like me for suggesting this but one option is to get up a little earlier, say 10 minutes. OK, I can see you are getting ready to throw the frying pan at me. So how about this? I know someone who found themselves in a similar situation to you. What they do is to lay out the breakfast dishers and cereals boxes before they go to bed. This skims a few minutes off the breakfast preparation time in the morning, time that can be spent actually eating breakfast. It serves as a reminder each morning to have something for breakfast, too. If your children are sitting down to eat breakfast, are you really not able to sit and eat breakfast with them?*

22

Lunch boxes

What's in your lunch box today? What do you mean you don't know? Breakfast might be the most important meal of the day, but you shouldn't ignore lunch.

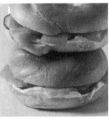

The high-paced pressure of modern life means that lunch is often forgotten. You've been working throughout the day only to find that when you finally stop for a break, it's suppertime.

This happens more often than you really care to admit. It's a tragedy of our times that more and more people are missing out on lunch. As a result of this what happens is you snack, usually on foods that offer short-term rewards but which are unhealthy and are not kind to your blood pressure. Even if you do have some lunch there's a good chance it will be a working one. If you're lucky the lunch is in a fine restaurant. However, it's more likely that you are sitting in a meeting room, a plate of quartered sandwiches from a local deli wilting on the table and a pot that threatens to burn your hand every time you try to release the brown beverage from its unique dispensing mechanism. There may even be a life-giving, and burn-soothing, jug of water standing to attention next to them. At least you have some chance of getting a little pleasure from lunch this way. There's not much hope, though, if you are sitting in front of the computer screen, juggling the sandwich in

Here's an idea for you...

Set a time when you and your colleagues have lunch together. Each day everyone brings one item of food, enough for everyone to have some, and you have an office picnic or buffet. If possible have it away from the working area or outside. In time it will become an established routine to stop work for lunch. Since everyone will be taking part you will feel less pressure to continue working through lunch.

one hand and the drink in the other as you try to type, move the mouse, or talk on the phone. Sound familiar? Well, you're certainly not alone. Desk lunches are taking over.

So are lunches on the go. Pacing from one meeting to the next, trying to talk on your cell with a crusty roll stuffed in your mouth—at least you're having lunch, but it certainly isn't a good way to have it. You will not be able to digest it properly, which means you'll soon be feeling uncomfortable. And you'll be stressed at the same time. Such a waste when eating is one of the real pleasures in life. What you are eating is probably extremely unhealthy, too. All that saturated fat, salt, and calories will not be doing your blood pressure any good at all.

We often blame modern-day living for sucking up all our time, but missing lunch may have become a habit much earlier in our lives. Think back to your school days and trading your lunch snack for sports cards. I know someone who decided that if he went without lunch he could save his lunch money to spend on something he really wanted, like a new football or a pair of the latest sneakers. This may have been a good financial strategy but it left his health strategy somewhat empty. It left his stomach empty as well.

You've seen the phrase "out to lunch." It used to appear in shop windows. And no, it didn't mean that the person was a few sandwiches short of a picnic. It meant that they had actually gone out to lunch. It's not often seen now since, like many businesses, shops no

Worried whether your lunch is good for your blood pressure? Salt is the main problem here, so sift through IDEA 25, *The salt of the earth.*

Try another idea...

longer close for lunch. You don't need a sign, although you could make one if it helps. Just leaving your workstation, switching off your cell phone, and spending half an hour having a lunch break will leave you refreshed and efficient on your return. Oh, you'll be a nicer person to work with as well. By having lunch somewhere different each day you won't get bored of the same old routine and slip back into unhealthy habits.

If you're eating lunch while reading this, then I'll let you off. After all, hopefully you are in a relaxed spot enjoying both the food and the book.

"My body is like breakfast, lunch, and dinner. I don't think about it, I just have it."
ARNOLD SCHWARZENEGGER

Defining idea...

How did it go?

Q   I like going for lunch with colleagues, but how can I stop them from just talking about work?

A   *If you decide to continue having lunch with them you may need to lay down some ground rules. Let them know that lunchtime is a work-free zone. This means no work-related conversation, phone calls, or report reading. If this is likely to disrupt your harmonious working relationship, then why not follow the advice of the well-known quiz program and phone a friend, and arrange to have lunch with them? You'll be helping yourself and your friend, too, if they are not in the habit of having a lunch break either. Just be careful not to spend the time unloading about work.*

Q   I'm finding that it's a little expensive eating out every day. Any tips?

A   *Buying lunch from work cafeterias or local food stores can be expensive, especially if you work in a city. Making your own packed lunch is often cheaper, and you can have what you like, so long as it's good for your blood pressure. Sandwiches made with whole grain bread, chicken, lean meat, or fish and plenty of salad are good. Use low-fat mayonnaise or avoid it altogether. Mustard, black pepper, or pickles will add flavor. Try a tuna or chicken salad, or have some pasta. If you usually have lunch with a colleague, take turns preparing lunch for each other. It's often less expensive if you make lunch for two, rather than two people making it separately.*

23

Bottoms up

A little drop won't kill you, it may even do you some good. Pull up a chair and find out how drinking alcohol can affect your blood pressure.

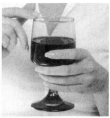

"A little bit of what you like does you good." It's true. So why when we hear it said is this phrase invariably being used by our inner defense lawyer?

With regards to drinking alcohol, we really should be able to confidently raise our glass and say, "Good health." Times have indeed changed for alcoholic drinks. They're now up there in the premier division with the great and the good since research suggests that a moderate amount may help us to keep healthy. It can protect the heart, for example, and of course one of the reasons for making sure blood pressure doesn't become high is also to protect the heart from harm. A moderate amount of alcohol can protect against having a stroke, too—the kind that affects the brain, that is, not the kind that results from an alcohol-induced lack of inhibition and poor judgment.

Ah, I hear you say, so if a little is good for me, a lot must be even better! Sadly not. That was certainly the cry when the news about the benefits of drinking alcohol

Here's an idea for you... **For the next week, keep a record of all the alcoholic drinks you consume. At the end of the week total up how many drinks you have had. This will tell you just how much you really drink each week and whether you are helping or harming your blood pressure. Cheers!**

started to seep into the media. Men and women everywhere could be heard saying, or rather slurring, "I s'heard it (deep breath in) on the news. It'sh good for me. Dat's why I'sh drinking this you seeee," before falling down and suffering one of the many harms that drinking too much alcohol brings.

Drinking large amounts of alcohol will cause your blood pressure to rise. Why this happens isn't clear, but it does. Drinking large amounts of alcohol also contributes to weight gain, and this certainly can cause a rise in blood pressure. On the other hand, drinking small amounts doesn't increase blood pressure.

But how small is small and how much is too much? One of the most irritating answers a doctor gets given to the question how much do you drink is, "Oh, normal amounts." I know of people for whom a normal amount is just one beer a week, whereas others may believe that drinking this amount every couple of hours is normal. There was a time when a normal amount for a friend of mine meant less than two-thirds of a pint of cider. Any more than this and he would be singing like a leprechaun on acid before passing out on the floor. Then there are those at the other end of the scale who can drink a fish under the table with no visible effects.

In the past, doctors simply preached "everything in moderation." Helpful—not! What this actually meant was that the medical profession had no idea how much alcohol was safe to drink. Some doctors would go that little bit further and say, "So long as you don't drink as much as me then you should be all right!"

Flavonoids in red wine are believed to protect the blood vessels from harm. IDEA 24, *Say hello to antioxidants*, introduces more body protectors.

Try another idea...

However, now there's very clear advice as to what is a safe amount to drink. For men, it's up to two servings a day, for women it's one serving a day, where a serving is half a pint of ordinary strength beer or lager, one small glass of wine, or one shot of spirits. Those who have high blood pressure are usually advised to limit their alcohol consumption to no more than fourteen servings a week for men, and no more than seven servings a week for women. And if the fear of high blood pressure isn't enough to encourage someone to reduce the amount of alcohol they consume, try telling them that just as tennis elbow doesn't only affect tennis players, beer belly doesn't only affect beer drinkers.

"All excess is ill, but drunkenness is of the worst sort. It spoils health, dismounts the mind, and unmans men. It reveals secrets, is quarrelsome, lascivious, impudent, dangerous, and bad."
WILLIAM PENN

Defining idea...

101

How did it go?

Q **This week was an unusual one for me—it was a heavier one as far as alcohol was concerned. Honest. How can I get an accurate assessment of my intake?**

A *If you think that the week you've chosen was a particularly "heavy" one, let's say that you went to a party or two, or had more liquid lunches than normal, then try keeping the record over, say, four weeks. This will give you a more accurate, and possibly more sobering, indication of your alcohol consumption.*

Q **My job takes me to many business meetings where there's always plenty of alcohol. How can I avoid the booze on these occasions?**

A *Ah yes, the "it's out of my control" excuse. Just because the alcohol is there doesn't mean that you have to drink it. Stop kidding yourself. Try alternating alcoholic drinks with non-alcoholic ones the next time you're in one of these meetings. If you also include some fruit juice you'll be working toward reaching your target of five portions of fruits and vegetables each day, and your daily eight glasses of water requirement. You'll be sharper and more focused, which in business is what helps you keep on top.*

Q **I've had more than is healthy for me. It was a bit of a shock to be honest. What should I do?**

A *Try this: For each drink you consume write down the number of servings as a running total, just as a bartender might keep a tab for you. This will tell you just how quickly in the week you leave the safe alcohol consumption zone and start to put your blood pressure, and other parts of your body, at risk.*

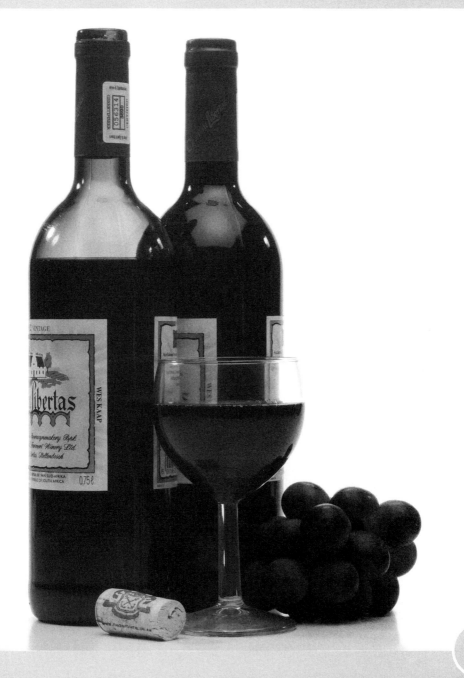

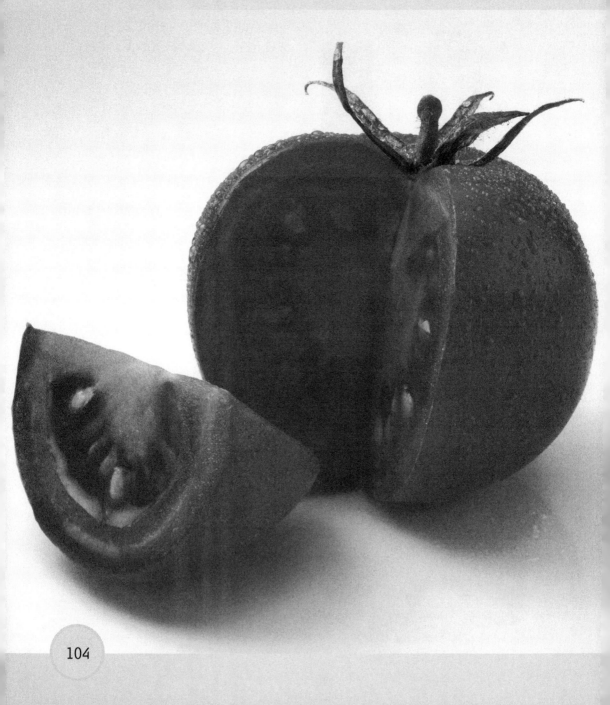

24

Say hello to antioxidants

These little housekeepers spend their time mopping up the troublemakers inside us. Unlike mother's little helpers, these will help keep your body in tip-top shape.

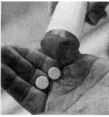

You've heard the saying, only two things are certain in life, death and taxes. Well, you can't stop the tax man from calling, but you can delay death knocking on your door.

In order for your healthy working body to stay healthy and working, it needs to break down nutrients. This is how your body gets the energy it needs. As part of this process, which to be fair is invariably very efficient, by-products are formed. These are called free radicals and result from many chemical processes within and among cells. As in many things in life, and indeed in health, it's not good to have too much of something. A surplus of free radicals can wreak havoc within your body, like a room full of gremlins that have been left unsupervised. These free radicals contribute to blood vessel damage, which may result in heart attacks and strokes, and damage to cells that may cause cancer.

Free radicals are also created following exposure to environmental factors such as ionizing radiation from sunshine, ozone and nitrous oxide from car exhausts, and

Make a list of seven brightly colored fruits and vegetables. Each day of the week make sure you have at least one of them. Have a cup of green tea every day, too, so you get a good amount of all the beneficial antioxidants.

cigarette smoke. Oh yes, there are lots of sources of the little devils to threaten the balance and harmony of your body's well-being.

This is where antioxidants come to the rescue. They are the body's superheroes. They counteract these free radicals by binding to them, transforming them into non-harmful compounds and repairing any cell damage. Put simply, you could also call them the body's housekeeper since they do the "mopping up." The best-known antioxidants are vitamins A, C, and E, often called ACE. Others that are coming off the subs bench and making a name for themselves include selenium and lycopene.

However, the reality is that much of the food eaten these days is processed and lacking in essential vitamins and minerals. So the equation isn't looking too healthy, is it? If you have too many free radicals but not enough antioxidants to deactivate them, then you're left with a body that is vulnerable to free radical damage.

So where do you get these little gems known as antioxidants? It's back to the fruits and vegetables, an excellent source of antioxidants. The most deeply or brightly colored fruits and vegetables, such as tomatoes, red peppers, blueberries, cranberries, and carrots, have particularly high concentrations. So does red wine and green tea, both of which are packed with antioxidants called flavonoids. It's because fresh fruits and vegetables are such good sources of antioxidants that eating five portions of fruits and vegetables a day is recommended. Turmeric, grape seed, ginkgo biloba, and pine bark extracts also have antioxidant benefits.

The $64,000 question (because you're worth it...) is can antioxidants prevent aging? Well, the jury is out on this one but currently the feelings are that the verdict is likely to be no. Although they may not be able to stop the process of aging, antioxidants may be able to slow it down. It's believed that they can delay death, of course, by reducing the risk of heart disease and some cancers.

We talk a lot about blood pressure, usually the two blood pressure figures. Try IDEA 1, *Pump up the volume*, to find out what these really mean.

Try another idea...

Now these antioxidants may not directly affect your blood pressure but think about why doctors get so worked up about blood pressure in the first place. It's because high blood pressure is a risk factor for heart attacks and strokes. A lack of antioxidants is another risk factor. So although antioxidants may be a different player, they're on the same team trying to score in the same goal. And that goal is to stay alive and keep on playing, and not end up taking an early out.

"Keeping your body healthy is an expression of gratitude to the whole cosmos—the trees, the clouds, everything."
THICH NHAT HANH

Defining idea...

How did it go?

Q   I find it difficult to eat enough fruits and vegetables. Any tips?

A   *If you're not in the habit of eating fruits and vegetables there are lots of things that can help. For starters, you need to put the fruits and vegetables where you can see them. Remember, if something is out of sight, then it is really going to be out of mind. Next, these foods must be accessible: Make sure that they are left around your home and workplace where you can reach for them easily. Start by making a point of eating one piece of fruit each day, and then gradually build up. You probably don't need any advice on drinking red wine, so why not have some fruit each time you drink a glass?*

Q   Can I get what I need from a supplement?

A   *In the long run relying on a supplement is probably not the best way of getting the antioxidants you need. In fruits and vegetables there are many different nutrients and chemicals that do not appear in supplements. These additional nutrients are thought to work together, in partnership with nutrients from other foods, to benefit and protect the body. In the short-term, however, taking a supplement will at least give you some of the antioxidants you need while you are establishing the routine of eating a variety of fresh fruits and vegetables every day.*

25

The salt of the earth

For centuries salt has been enjoyed and seen as a sign of hospitality and wealth. But you know what they say, "Too much of a good thing..." Well, salt is no exception.

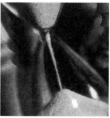

Traditionally salt was offered as a gift or in payment. A host showed how much he valued his guests by placing salt on the table.

Even today when a table is laid before a meal you can almost guarantee that the salt-shaker will be there, often taking center stage. But nowadays it's there to enhance flavor, or through habit.

We now know that a high intake of salt is linked to high blood pressure, which in turn increases the risk of heart attacks and strokes. Salt is made up of sodium and chloride and it's the sodium that's bad for us. Small amounts of sodium, however, are needed by the body if it is to function properly. Muscle contraction, nerve impulse transmission, and the maintenance of correct water balance in the body all need sodium.

Most of us routinely consume far more salt than we need. In fact, it's estimated that, on average, adults have around 9 grams a day, possibly even as much as 12 grams a day. This is far more than the current recommendation of no more than 6 grams a day, which is roughly equivalent to a level teaspoon of the stuff.

Here's an idea for you... **Check food labels to see which foods are high and low in sodium. As a rule of thumb foods containing 0.1 gram or less of sodium per 100 grams are fine. Foods containing 0.5 gram or more of sodium per 100 grams are not. By doing this you'll get into the habit of recognizing which foods are good, and not so good, for blood pressure.**

If you're feeling uncomfortable reading this, relax. I'm not trying to add salt to your wound. It's really not your fault that you enjoy salt so much. Most people grew up with salt being added to cooking. Once served, the automatic response was to add salt to the food on the plate. It just happened, there was no question about it, because it was normal practice. And like most people you enjoyed and became accustomed to the taste.

If there's one thing you can do to get your blood pressure into the safety zone, it's to reduce the amount of salt you eat. One of the simplest ways of doing this is not to add salt to food when cooking—vegetables, rice, potatoes, and pasta, for example. Another quick and easy step is not to add salt to food at the table. Move the saltshaker from the table if necessary, or ask someone to hide it.

Reducing your intake of salt in this way will certainly help to keep blood pressure at a safe level. But it probably will not be enough. The problem is that up to 80 percent of the salt we consume each day is hidden in food. Prepackaged food, takeout meals, canned beans, processed meats (sausages, bacon, pâté), and premade sandwiches are just a few of the guilty parties. Some breakfast cereals (and you thought these were healthy, didn't you?) contain as much salt as Atlantic seawater (1 gram sodium/100 grams). So it's best to eat less of these high-salt foods in addition to not cooking with salt or adding it to meals.

Potassium can help reduce salt in the body, and bananas are a good source. So try out IDEA 27, Have a banana.

Try another idea...

Choose foods that are labeled as having reduced sodium or salt content. Eat fresh meat and fish instead of processed varieties, and eat more fruits and vegetables since the potassium in these helps the body to lose sodium. Sauces, pickles, and mayonnaise tend to be high in salt, too, so limit how much of these you have.

It's helpful to try to keep a tally of the amount of salt you consume each day. But beware, food labels can be misleading. They often list the sodium content of the foods, which is much less than the salt content. To get the salt content of food you need to multiply the sodium figure by 2.5—for example, if the sodium content on the packet is 0.8 gram, then the salt content is actually 2 grams. If your daily tally is greater than 6 grams of salt, or greater than 2.4 grams of sodium, then you're having too much.

"A little more moderation would be good. Of course, my life hasn't exactly been one of moderation."
DONALD TRUMP

Defining idea...

How did it go?

Q   I tried leaving the salt out of my cooking, but how come all my food tastes dull now?

A   *This is normal. Taste buds get used to the salt in foods. Many people find that food tastes bland when they stop using so much salt. Before very long your taste buds will become more sensitive and adapt to the new flavors. In fact, this usually only takes a matter of weeks. This means you'll start enjoying the real flavor of the food and you'll probably find that high-salt foods taste unpleasant. Also, try to eat low-salt versions of the processed foods that are difficult to avoid, such as breakfast cereals and bread. Compare food products and choose the ones with less sodium.*

Q   I love salt. How else can I get flavor?

A   *There are many ways to add flavor to food without adding to your blood pressure. Try using garlic, chili, herbs, or black pepper to flavor food instead of salt. Although it's best not to use salt at all, if you can't go without it, using something that contains less sodium, and which also contains potassium, will at least provide you with some benefit. Check with your doctor before using a salt alternative if you have kidney disease or other medical problems, or are taking medication, as a large increase in potassium may cause you problems. Rock, sea, and garlic salt are basically the same as ordinary salt, so don't cheat by using these as an alternative!*

26

Gimme five

**Let's find out how a fruit and veggie high-five can help
your blood pressure get down.**

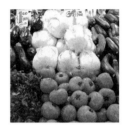

Remember when you were growing up,
and your mom or dad would say, "Eat your
greens, cabbage will make your hair curly,
carrots will make you see in the dark."

Experts now recommend that each and every one of us should eat at least five
portions of fruits and vegetables every day. And not because the food mountains
need reducing either. We may have thought that our parents, grandparents,
aunties, and uncles were trying to punish us, but they weren't. It turns out that the
wise ones in our family were basically right.

It's true that an apple a day helps keep the doctor away. In fact, an apple, a banana, a
glass of 100 percent fruit juice, a handful of dried apricots, and three tablespoons of
green peas a day, for example, will keep the doctor, the nurse, and the surgeon away.
It will even keep the undertaker away—at least for a while. Eating just five portions
of fruits and vegetables every day reduces the risk of becoming overweight, suffering

Here's an idea for you...

Put pieces of fruit at different places around your home and office, so you can see them and they're within easy reach. Put some on your desk, by your computer, and next to where you sit to watch TV. This will help you eat five portions a day, and help you to lose weight, too, since you won't be eating so many unhealthy snacks.

diabetes, heart disease, or stroke, and reduces the risk of developing certain cancers, to name but a few of the many health benefits.

Five portions a day is not much, is it? Perhaps not, but as far as the body is concerned it will do, thank you very much. Those five portions usually provide all the vitamins and minerals the body needs. Yes, a multivitamin and mineral supplement will also provide all the recommended daily amounts (RDA), but apparently, like in most aspects of life, having the real thing is just better.

So how many portions have you had today? Probably not five. But don't feel bad, you'd be in the majority. Very few people actually manage to eat more than two or three portions a day. If our parents had said cabbage will make your hair grow, rather than it will make it curly, then men in particular would be stuffing themselves with cabbage every day. There would be the gas to contend with, but hey, no pain no gain.

That at least would be a start. However, variety is the spice of life, and it's variety that's important. When you're out shopping, you probably buy the same fruit and vegetables. It's a comfort thing. But you wouldn't keep drinking the same wine, so why stick to the same fruits and veggies every time? Take a good look around the supermarket or farmers' market (the latter are an endangered species: Try to see one in its natural habitat while you still can) next time you're doing the weekly shopping. There's so much choice, and the food shelves are just bursting with new flavors all the time.

One of the problems we're all faced with is the abundance of convenience foods and snacks. You're at your desk, you're feeling hungry, or you're bored and just want to eat somehing. Recognize the feeling? Yes, sure you do. And so you reach for a snack bar or a cookie or some chocolate. Why? Because it's there, just waiting for you. You can see it, you want it, and it tastes good. Often we'll just reach out and eat whatever's there, without even thinking about it. Certainly without enjoying the experience. We're on autopilot. Eyes fixed on the television or movie screen, hands reaching around for food. It's a reflex.

I know someone who took advantage of his habit of always reaching into the cookie jar by reversing the roles. He put cookies and snacks in the fruit bowl and put fruit around the cookie jar. This way when autopilot carried him to the cookie jar he found fruit. Before long he was raising his hand in the air and saying, "Gimme five."

While we're on the subject of fruit, take a bite out of IDEA 20, *Apples and pears*.

Try another idea...

"Changing our diet is something we choose to do, not something we are forced to do. Instead of dreading it, try saying, 'Here's another thing I get to do to help myself. Great!' "
GREG ANDERSON, author

Defining idea...

115

How did it go?

Q **I'm doing OK at home but when I go for a coffee break at work there are always open packages of cookies around, and you've guessed it, I have to have one, or two, or... How do I stop this?**

A *Someone buys the cookies, yes? And I expect that you contribute to the kitty? Try asking the person who buys the coffee, tea, milk, and cookies if they could buy some fruit, too. I'm sure that there's a choice of milk—full, two percent, skim—since everyone has his or her own tastes. You probably have a choice of coffee with caffeine or without. I've worked in places where there are five or six different types of tea as well. So there's no reason why there shouldn't be a choice of snacks. Tell your colleagues what you're trying to do, they'll probably want to do it, too, particularly if they hear that it may help them lose weight.*

Q **I've bought different fruits and vegetables but I still seem to come back to eating the same old ones. How I can I break out of this rut?**

A *Instead of going to your usual supermarket, buy your fruits and vegetables for the week from the local market. Farmers' markets, for example, are a tremendous place for getting bargains since fruits and vegetables in season are usually less expensive. Healthy food and financial benefit: A real double whammy! If you don't have a market nearby, then try choosing at least one different type of fruit or vegetable—one that you wouldn't usually buy— each time you go to the supermarket.*

27

Have a banana

Possibly the nation's favorite fruit, the list of benefits from bananas keeps on growing. Although you may slip up on the skin, the fruit can help your blood pressure slip down.

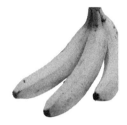

They're bright yellow, delicious to eat, and they're a funny shape. You can't help but smile when you hold one. In fact, hold a banana horizontally and it'll smile back at you.

You're probably smiling now as you read this. But it's true. Bananas are now believed to be able to help lower blood pressure. That's right, and it's official, too. The US Food and Drug Administration has given permission to banana producers to claim that eating bananas can reduce the risk of developing high blood pressure and strokes.

So eating a couple of bananas each day, as part of a healthy diet that contains plenty of different fruits and vegetables, could help keep high blood pressure at bay. Research has shown that just eating two bananas a day can reduce blood pressure by 10 percent. Bananas contain lots of potassium, which helps the body to lose sodium. And it's sodium that causes blood pressure levels to rise, which is why a reduction

Here's an idea for you...

Eat two bananas a day. Have one for breakfast and one as a mid-afternoon snack. This way if you are someone who doesn't usually have breakfast you'll find how easy it is to do so. The mid-afternoon snack banana will help you overcome that end-of-the-day sluggish feeling. And you'll be helping to keep your blood pressure healthy, without any effort.

in salt intake is generally recommended. Now, I'm not saying you should just live on bananas. It's important to eat a wide variety of fruits and vegetables. In fact, just as a little potassium can help, too much can cause problems, particularly if someone has kidney disease or is already taking medication to lower blood pressure, for example. So don't overdo the bananas, and check with your doctor if you're uncertain about anything.

The story doesn't stop here. The banana feel-good factor means we are less likely to turn to those unhealthy snacks, or worship the false gods of fast food and alcohol. You can't honestly tell me that you haven't felt your mood lift when you hold one in your hand. On the subject of mood lifting, bananas are also a good source of tryptophan, a natural mood enhancer. Since bananas contain good amounts of vitamins C, A, B$_6$, potassium, and magnesium, which soften the effects of nicotine withdrawal, bananas can help if you're trying to give up smoking.

A single banana counts as one of the five portions of fruits and vegetables we should all be eating each day. It's full of carbohydrates and so is a compact source of energy that should help us exercise. Why else would top golfers like Greg Norman, Nick Faldo, and Tiger Woods, and top tennis stars like Tim Henman and Andre Agassi eat them as a mid-game snack?

Bananas make a great start to the day. Try IDEA 21, *Come on, it's time for breakfast*, to see what else gets you off on the right foot.

Try another idea...

Bananas really are the perfect snack. They are easy to eat and are not messy. They come in a biodegradable wrapper (that can be used to treat plantar warts, by the way). They taste and smell good, and they do you good. What more could you ask for? They're not expensive either. Children love bananas, it's one of the fruits that is easy to get them to eat. What's more, a medium-size banana has only half a gram of fat.

Although you may find this hard to believe, some people do actually become a little bored eating bananas. To overcome this think of all the different ways you can eat a couple of bananas each day. To start you off here are a few suggestions: banana sandwich, banana custard, sliced banana added to breakfast cereal or oatmeal. Try sticking one unpeeled onto your grill in the summer. Yum! Once again, it's best to eat a wide variety of fruits and vegetables, not just one type.

"You have to stay in shape. My grandmother, she started walking five miles a day when she was 60. She's 97 today and we don't know where the hell she is."
ELLEN DEGENERES

Defining idea...

119

How did it go?

Q   What can I do if I don't like the texture of bananas?

A   Try making a banana smoothie either on it's own or with some other fruit added, such as strawberries or raspberries. This is a great energy-giving way to start the day, and very refreshing later in the day, too. Blend apple juice, strawberries, and a couple of bananas. Add some honey if you think it needs sweetening. Delicious. You can also slice a banana and place the slices on a piece of toast. Firmly smooth the banana into the toast and, presto, it's ready to eat.

Q   I really don't like bananas. Are there any alternatives?

A   Well, how about eating some other potassium-rich foods like oranges and orange juice, grapefruit juice, potatoes, tomatoes, peaches, papaya, passion fruit, dried apricots, peas, beans, spinach, parsnips, and legumes? There are plenty of choices so you don't have to miss out on the blood pressure lowering benefits of foods.

Q   Why are bananas so good for an energy boost?

A   They provide a release of energy gradually over a period of time. This means that you don't get the energy highs and lows that candy and cookies can cause—you know, the ones where immediately after eating you feel energized only to find yourself nodding off a few hours later. In fact, eating two bananas can give you enough energy for a 90-minute workout. That's why so many sports professionals eat them.

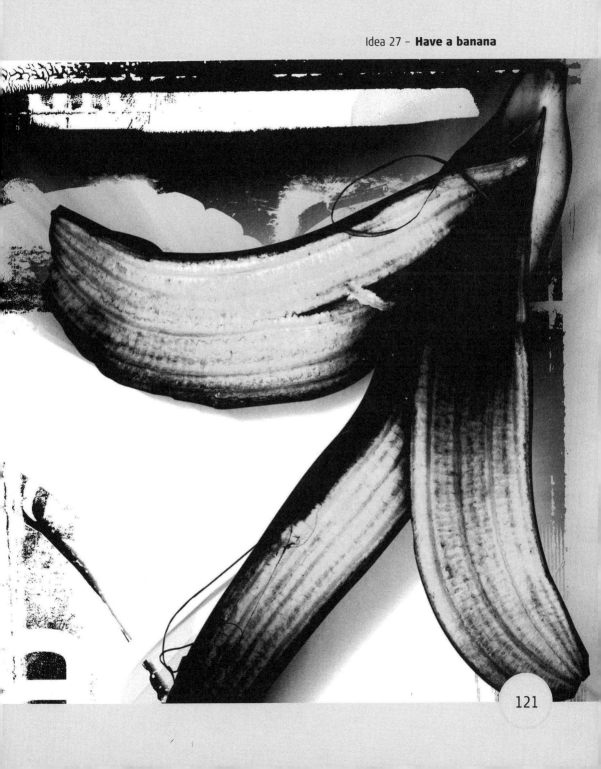

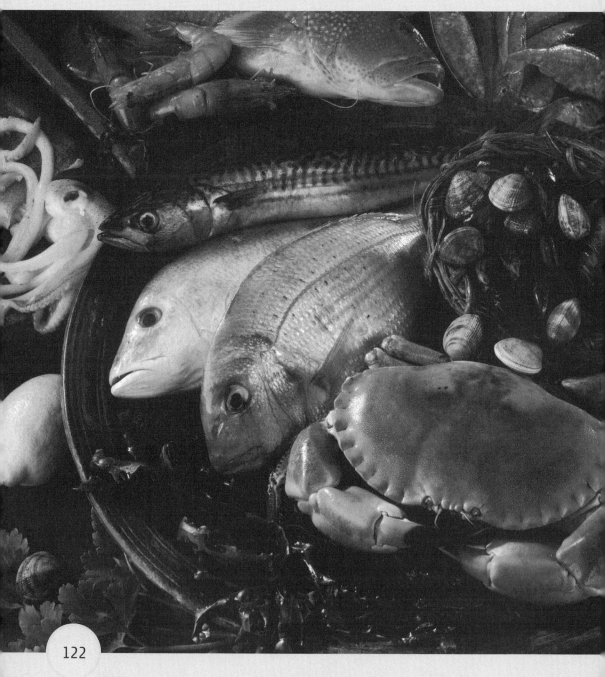

28

Fish like the Eskimos

The Eskimo populations of Alaska and Greenland eat a high-fat diet but have low levels of heart disease. So what's the answer to this conundrum? It's in the fish.

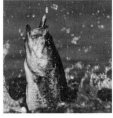

The deepwater fish eaten as a staple by these populations are rich in omega-3 fatty acids, and researchers discovered that this particular type of fatty acid protects the heart.

There is now good scientific evidence that eating oily fish reduces the risk of death from heart disease because they're a good source of omega-3 polyunsaturated fatty acids. White fish also contain these fatty acids, but at much lower levels than oily fish.

Omega-3 fatty acids work by reducing the "stickiness" of the blood, making it less likely to clot. They also protect the arteries from becoming damaged. In addition they prevent the heart from beating irregularly, they lower levels of fats called triglycerides that are associated with heart disease, and what's more they may help lower your blood pressure, too.

Here's an idea for you...

Experts now recommend that people eat at least two portions of fish a week, one of which should be oily. During the next week have one portion of oily fish. The following week have two portions of fish, one oily and one white fish such as cod, haddock, or flounder.

You may have seen ads for fish oils, essential fatty acids, and omega-3s. These terms generally all refer to the same thing. What's in a name, after all? What is important is that these essential fish oils help to look after your heart and stop you from getting lost in the deep blue sea. They are called essential because your body can't make them; they have to be obtained from your diet.

These omega-3 fatty acids don't just look after the heart. They are also important for the development of the central nervous system in babies, before and after they are born. There is some evidence suggesting that if women eat oily fish when they are pregnant and when breast-feeding, this helps their baby's development.

Compared to the Eskimos, you don't have to work hard for your fish. No standing on an ice floe pretending not to be polar bear food. Your fish are caught, packaged, and sometimes even delivered to your doorstep. All you have to do is eat them. Oh, you may have to cook the fish or remove it from the can but that's hardly difficult, is it?

Most of us don't eat fish very often. It's not clear why, we just don't. Maybe it's the appearance. Having the head on the plate isn't always the most appealing thing to look at, or to have looking back at you. Maybe it's the fear of the bones. After all, we were all taught the dangers of fish bones and to be wary of them. Perhaps it's simply that with the skin and bones to deal with fish is sometimes classed as a hard-work food. Who knows? However, this is where eating fish and gaining the benefits of oily fish becomes easy.

Mackerel, salmon, fresh tuna, sardines, herring, and trout all contain high levels of omega-3 fatty acids. Now before you sit back and rest on your laurels, pay attention. You'll notice it's fresh tuna that's included in the list. Tinned or canned tuna doesn't count. I know, it's not fair, but it doesn't. Why not? Although canned tuna is delicious, and we love it with salads, in sandwiches, and with pasta, I'm sorry but during the canning process the amount of omega-3 fats is reduced. So although it's tasty and good for us in other ways, tinned or canned tuna does not count toward our weekly requirement of oily fish.

But all the other oily fish count whether they are fresh or come out of a can. And you don't have to eat the same fish each week. Although you'll get all the omega-3s that your body needs this way, you're likely to become bored. So try a different fish each week, and try eating it in different ways.

Obviously a key part of a healthy lifestyle is the food we eat. Try IDEA 30, *Living it up in the Med*, to see why living the Mediterranean way is so good for you.

Try another idea...

"To safeguard one's health at the cost of too strict a diet is a tiresome illness indeed."
FRANÇOIS DE LA ROCHEFOUCAULD

Defining idea...

How did it go?

Q I don't eat fish. How can I get more omega-3 in my diet?

A Don't despair. Many other foods contain omega-3 fatty acids. Although not as good as oily fish, the following plants and foods contain omega-3 fatty acids: dark leafy green vegetables, cereals, peanuts, almonds, pecans, walnuts, rapeseed or canola oil, soy oil, beans, and tofu. If these don't interest you, or you are worried that you may not get enough omega-3 fatty acids, then good supplements are easily available from pharmacists and health food stores.

Q So if oily fish is good for us, shouldn't we eat as much as possible?

A It's recommended that everyone should eat at least two portions of fish a week, one of which should be oily fish. A portion is around 140 grams. There are limits for some people, however. At the time of writing it's recommended that girls and women of childbearing age, or who are already pregnant, or who are breast-feeding should not eat more than two portions of oily fish each week. Men, and women who are not going to become pregnant, can eat up to four portions of oily fish a week. The reasoning behind this advice is that oily fish contain certain chemicals that although unlikely to effect health in the short-term, if taken in high levels over a long period of time may prove harmful.

29

To supplement or not to supplement?

That is the question. Could a supplement assist in the quest for healthy blood pressure? There's only one way to find out.

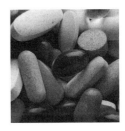

There is much debate about the use of supplements in keeping blood pressure within the safety zone. It's the same with any idea. Someone makes a claim, and research either supports or dismisses it.

Proponents will argue that herbal, homeopathic, and nutritional remedies have been used for years without problems and are therefore beneficial and safe. Conventionalists will counter this by saying that these therapies have not been studied so it is not possible to say whether they work or are safe. The debate rages on and while scientists research the effects of various supplements on blood pressure, around the globe high blood pressure is on the rise, and so is the billion-dollar supplement market.

Here's an idea for you... **Provided your doctor has given you the OK, try taking your preferred supplement. Garlic and fish oil, for example, may both help lower blood pressure. Check your blood pressure before, and after one, two, and three months of taking the supplement. If your blood pressure becomes lower, then taking the supplement may have contributed to this.**

Research is ongoing, and only in time will we know which supplements, and in what dose, may help to keep blood pressure firmly in the safety zone. In the meantime, let's take a sensible approach.

A supplement is precisely that, a supplement. It's not intended to replace or be an alternative to a healthy lifestyle. It would be nice if it were. We could then all eat, drink, and be merry, and our heart truly would be content. But for the moment this is fantasy. Salt reduction, exercise, and keeping to an ideal weight are some of the most effective ways we can lower our blood pressure to healthy levels. Some supplements may help keep blood pressure healthy and, importantly, if our diet has any deficiences, they can fill in the gaps, as a dietary insurance policy.

Research has demonstrated that low levels of potassium are linked to high blood pressure. Therefore getting additional potassium into the body can help to prevent high blood pressure. But, and it's a big but, too much potassium can have disastrous effects on the body, so it's recommended that potassium be acquired through diet rather than via supplements. So increasing the amount of potassium-rich foods you eat each day—e.g., bananas, peaches, green peppers, spinach, peas, watercress, papayas, and apricots—may be a good idea. You don't have to eat the same ones every day. Once you have gone through the list look on the Internet or in a nutrition guide and make a list of all the potassium-rich foods you can find. Then start working your way through those. Although potassium supplements are available, it's important to only take them if your doctor has approved and is supervising you doing this.

If you think about the A, B, C, as the Jackson's said, it really is as easy as one, two, three.

A is for advice. Always ask your doctor for advice before taking any supplement or herbal product, particularly if you have an existing medical condition or are already taking medication. While a supplement may help one health problem, it may worsen another. Some supplements interact with prescribed medication and can lessen or amplify the effect of the medicine. Supplements should not be used in place of medication that has been prescribed.

B is for buying. Choose an established and well-known brand. Although other brands may be cheaper, sometimes paying a little more really does mean that you get what you pay for. Your doctor or qualified nutritionist should be able to advise the appropriate dose for you to take. Start off with no more than a few months' supply because this is where C comes into play.

C is for checking your blood pressure. Do this monthly while you're on your chosen supplement. Remember, if you have changed your lifestyle in other beneficial ways in addition to taking a supplement, and your blood pressure is lowered, it will be difficult to know what was responsible for the improvement.

So until science confirms categorically whether certain supplements can help to keep blood pressure at a healthy level or not, remember, "first do no harm" and watch this space!

While you're in the mood for separating fact and fiction, try IDEA 33, *Challenge cholesterol*.

Try another idea...

"The higher your energy level, the more efficient your body. The more efficient your body, the better you feel and the more you will use your talent to produce outstanding results."
ANTHONY ROBBINS

Defining idea...

**Q   I've heard that taking a supplement of coenzyme Q10 can lower
blood pressure. Is this true?**

A   *Coenzyme Q10 is a natural substance produced by the body that helps speed
up vital metabolic processes. The body manufactures some coenzyme Q10
but also obtains it from foods such as fish, meat, green vegetables, and
nuts. Some studies have demonstrated that it can lower blood pressure in
those who have hypertension. Levels of coenzyme Q10 often start to fall
from around the age of twenty as the body produces less of it and less is
absorbed from the diet, and so many doctors recommend taking a
supplement of coenzyme Q10 from around the age of forty.*

**Q   I've heard that magnesium supplements can help to lower blood
pressure. Fact or fiction?**

A   *One minute the research says yes, it can help, the next minute research says
no, it can't. It has been suggested that a diet low in magnesium may cause
blood pressure to become high. Consequently taking a supplement or eating
more magnesium-rich foods such as green leafy vegetables, nuts, seeds,
whole grains, dried peas, and beans may help to lower blood pressure back
down into the safety zone.*

Q   What about vitamin C?

A   *Vitamin C is a powerful antioxidant and is believed to help keep the heart
healthy. Some studies have suggested that taking a supplement of vitamin C
may, among its other benefits, help to lower blood pressure.*

30

Living it up in the Med

OK, so you're not basking somewhere in the Mediterranean, you are lying on your sofa in your living room. This doesn't mean you can't enjoy a little of the Mediterranean lifestyle.

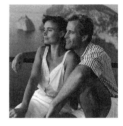

The sun is shining in the light blue sky. Sitting in the shade of a tree, you feel the cool breeze brushing against your face. Birds cheerfully sing in the distance.

The sound of waves soothes you as they gently lap in and out. You're in paradise.

A voice trespassing through your oasis announces two weeks, full board for only $499, including return flights and brings you back down to earth with a thump. You open your eyes to find that you drifted off to the Travel Channel.

You can still enjoy eating a Mediterranean diet wherever you are, and help your health in the bargain. And I'm not talking about losing weight so that you look great on the beach, although this may be a bonus. I'm talking about how the number of people with heart disease in Mediterranean countries is less than it is in the United States, even though the amount of fat eaten in Mediterranean countries

Here's an idea for you...

Watch TV vacation shows to learn about life in the Mediterranean. Jot down ideas and recipes to try out over the next week. Record the program if you like so you can watch it again. Oh, and if you see a competition to win a trip to the Mediterranean then enter it. You never know, you might get lucky.

is quite high. Since high blood pressure is a major risk factor for heart disease, a region that has low heart disease rates should be taken seriously.

If you have visited any of the many countries that border the Mediterranean you may be wondering how the diet can be good for you. The first thing you are likely to remember is how much oil there seemed to be. And you'd be right: Plenty of oil is used and consumed. Surely that can't be good? Well, actually, yes it can. Although olive oil is a source of fat, it's mostly monounsaturated fat, which is less likely to increase your cholesterol levels. In fact, research has shown that consuming olive oil can actually help lower cholesterol levels. Olive oil is believed also to contain antioxidants that discourage artery clogging. As usual, moderation is important here—olive oil is quite high in calories.

But think back to what else you ate while you were there. Lots of vegetables, fruit, bread, nuts, and seeds. You would have been offered fish, some of which would have been oily, which provides heart-protective omega-3 fatty acids that may also help to lower blood pressure. And you probably didn't eat as many dairy foods as you would at home. Dairy foods contain high levels of saturated fats, the fats that increase levels of bad cholesterol. Unless you went specifically looking for junk food, it's unlikely that you ate very much, if any, of this food that is likely to be high in saturated fats and salt. And don't forget the couple of glasses of wine that you enjoyed, which may help rather than hinder health when taken in moderation.

It's starting to make sense now, isn't it? You are seeing the forest for the trees. Around the world it is generally agreed that because the Mediterranean diet has more legumes, cereals, grains, pasta, nuts, olive oil, fruits, and vegetables, it is healthier than an American or Northern European diet.

While you're feeling so chilled and relaxed, before you slip into a siesta, check out IDEA 34, _Who let the stress out?_, since a little stress can be good for you, too.

Try another idea...

Generally speaking, the Mediterranean diet is simply a healthy diet. Lots of fruits and vegetables, a couple of portions of fish each week, not too many dairy products, and not too much red meat. It's the kind of diet any dietician would recommend that we all try to achieve. Rather than calling it a diet, it should really be called the Mediterranean lifestyle, since the reason behind heart disease levels being lower in these countries, and deaths from heart disease being lower, too, is not just because of the diet. Lifestyle factors such as more physical activity, better stress management, and extended social support systems also contribute to the health of the people there.

"If you need medical advice, let these three things be your physicians; a cheerful mind, relaxation from business, and a moderate diet."
SCHOLA SALERN

Defining idea...

How did it go?

Q   There don't seem to be any TV programs featuring the Mediterranean at the moment. Where can I get the info?

A   *Look on the Internet to get a feel for the lifestyle. Check out your local library for a Mediterranean recipe book. Over the course of the next week reproduce these meals at home a couple of times. Oh, and take your time over the meal: A leisurely pace helps digestion—something else those in the Mediterranean put to great effect.*

Q   Won't the food taste different if I use olive oil?

A   *I don't think you'll notice any difference. If, however, you don't like the flavor of the olive oil, when you cook with it add a few shavings of fresh garlic or some black pepper to the oil. You could also try cooking with rapeseed oil, since this contains monounsaturated fat, too.*

Q   I already cook with olive oil. Is there anything else I can do?

A   *Unless you visit places that specifically cater to tourists—you know, by basically offering food that is local, but adapted for foreign taste buds— you'll see that when bread is served it is accompanied by olive oil. Try this at home. Instead of spreading butter or margarine onto your bread, just trickle a few drops of olive oil onto it. By doing this you will still be livening up the bread, if you feel it needs this, but you'll be doing it with a healthier type of fat.*

31

Hey there, smoothie

If you're looking for a fantastic way to give your body and mind a healthy boost, then look no farther. Fruit smoothies are the way to go.

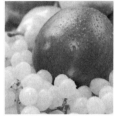

Take some fresh fruit and some low-fat yogurt and blend them together. That's basically all there is to it. It's so simple that even the most cooking-phobic among you can manage it.

What's even better about this is that you can choose which fruits you want to include. Throw in pretty much anything you like. That's the joy of smoothies; you can experiment to your heart's content. Make use of whatever fruit you have available; you probably have fruit lying around the kitchen anyway. You don't have to follow recipes to the letter; have fun trying out different combinations and inventing names for them. Nowadays you can get pretty much any fruit that you wish, since stores no longer only supply fruits that are in season.

It's quick, too. I know someone who was convinced that she didn't have time to make one for breakfast but she was pleasantly surprised. By the time you've made your morning cup of coffee, you'll have whipped up a smoothie that is ready for you to drink—if you haven't already swallowed it, that is. In fact, to speed the

Here's an idea for you...

Take one banana and cut it into chunks. Add five strawberries and ten raspberries. Blend these with three-quarters of a cup of skim or 2 percent milk or low-fat yogurt until the mixture is smooth. Take a moment to look at it and admire what you've created, and then drink it. Tastes good, doesn't it?

whole process up you can always prepare the fruit the night before and keep it in the refrigerator.

Smoothies are also perfect for conquering those mid-morning or mid-afternoon snack attacks the healthy way. You don't have to just have them at breakfast time. In the middle of the morning or the afternoon, when it's not quite time for lunch or dinner, they are just the thing. Since they are basically fruit, and packed with vitamins and minerals, they can help toward keeping blood pressure under control. You probably have a kettle or a coffeemaker at work. Why not suggest you also have a blender? Perhaps you could persuade everyone to chip in to buy one, so the whole office can join in the joy of smoothies.

If you should ever run out of ideas—and I'd be surprised if you did since you can combine just about anything—and you've exhausted recipe books and the Internet, here's something to try. Go into a store where they make and sell smoothies and ask them for their recipes. If they are reluctant to share these with you—as commercial establishments often are—just write down the combinations they list on their menus.

It's a good idea to have a fruit smoothie every day of the week. If you have one for breakfast, you'll be having at least one, and possibly more, of your daily five portions of fruits and vegetables, and you will start your day off on a high note.

While you're savoring your smoothie have a look at IDEA 29, *To supplement or not to supplement?*, to see whether you are getting enough of what your body needs.

Try another idea...

If you haven't made smoothies before, to begin with it's easier to make the same recipe every day. This way you get into the habit and will learn how much or how little of the ingredients you need. Then over the following weeks choose a different recipe, and so on. If you are becoming bored, then just experiment with different combinations and use a different recipe each day.

And if you want to spice things up in the evening or when you have friends around for a party, you can always add a little rum or vodka, or your favorite spirit, to your fruit smoothie to make the perfect healthy evening tipple. It might take a little experimentation before you achieve the perfect blend, but that shouldn't be an unpleasant experience.

So I'm sure that your mouth is already watering at the thought. If not, then your mind will be wanting to try out something that surely can't be as good as it's said to be.

"Drinking freshly made juices and eating enough whole foods to provide adequate fiber is a sensible approach to a healthful diet."
JAY KORDICH, author and juicing expert

Defining idea...

How did it go?

Q   I don't have a blender or food processor. How can I join the smoothie club?

A   *It would be easy to suggest that you buy one, but as with exercise equipment, it may sit there on your kitchen countertop gathering dust. Ask your friends if theirs is sitting idle and if you can borrow it. You may be doing them a favor. It is possible to make a smoothie without a blender or food processor. Doing it this way, however, means you are unlikely to get the same smooth consistency that you get with a blender. It also takes a little more effort on your part but that's OK because it will count as activity, so you are getting an extra bonus from the smoothie. To make a smoothie without the use of a blender start by placing soft-textured fruit—for example, strawberries or raspberries—in a bowl and mash them with a fork. Next, press these through a sieve into a large jug. Add the milk or yogurt and whisk until the mixture is frothy. Then enjoy it.*

Q   I've made a few smoothies now but they are a little bitter. Any tips for me?

A   *Try adding a little honey to the mixture. Bear in mind that if you use a sour or tart fruit it's a good idea to balance this out by adding a sweet fruit. Adding a few ice cubes makes it a very refreshing snack in warm weather, too.*

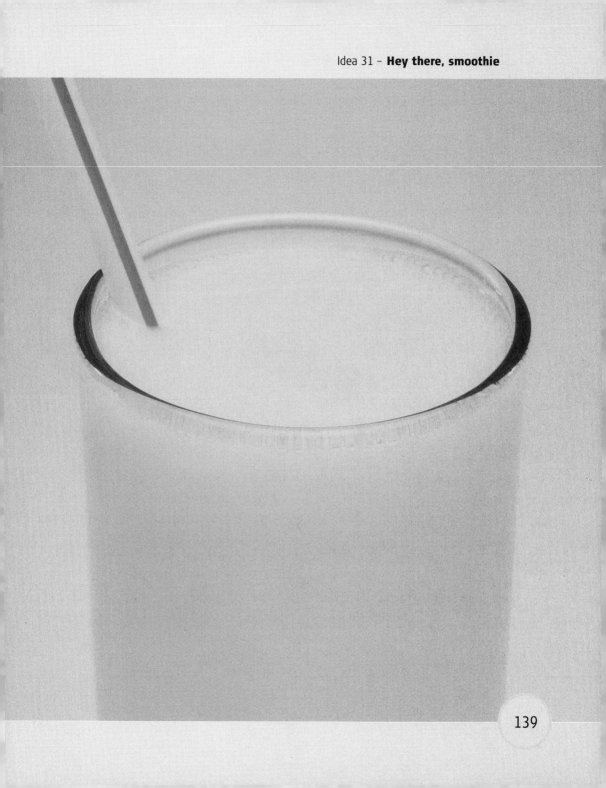

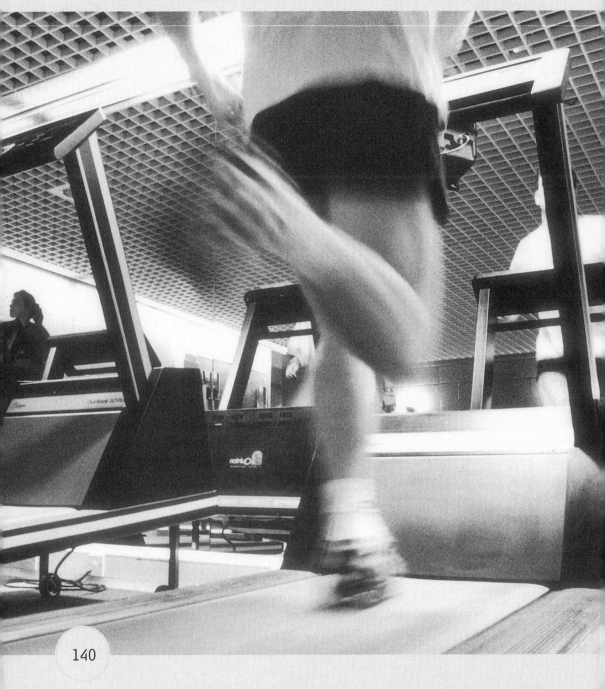

32

Drop some pounds

Fact: Losing weight is not easy. If it were simple there wouldn't be a new diet plan on the market almost every week. Fact: Losing weight is possible. And here's how.

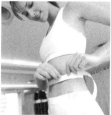

You saw the heading and thought, "Oh no, losing weight." In an instant you looked elsewhere along the list of other chapters and wanted to read a different one.

But you're still here, so well done! This page is probably the most thumbed but the least read. So far it is anyway. And that's exactly how it is with trying to lose weight. In your heart you know you have to, you've tried lots of times and got only so far, and then you've been frightened off and gone elsewhere. But all the while, it's been nagging at you.

Eating three meals a day, starting with breakfast, and eating healthy snacks in between if necessary, should keep your hunger at bay. Most people don't do this but still eat more food than ever before. The food eaten is often more unhealthy, too. One of the major factors that has contributed to the obesity crisis is the "all you can eat" and "buy one, get one free" offers that confront us wherever we go. We like to eat food; we also like to get a "good deal."

Here's an idea for you...

To lose weight become more active and try reducing your meal portion size. If you are cooking for yourself, cut your servings by around 25 percent. If eating out, try the children's meal, or if you're with a friend, then share a meal. This will reduce your calorie intake and you will feel satisfied rather than uncomfortable.

Inactivity is a growing problem and a major contributor to weight gain. On the way to work we sit on the bus, train, or in the car. At work we sit in front of the computer. Back home we fall onto the sofa in front of the TV, usually snacking. End result: obesity, which in turn increases our blood pressure. Lose some weight and your blood pressure will fall into the safety zone. In fact, you can lower your blood pressure by up to one point by just losing one pound of weight.

There is no quick fix to losing weight; it needs discipline and a little work. Yes, I know you lost weight when you did the "stand on one leg eating a doughnut diet," but you put the weight back on, didn't you? You will lose weight on most diets. That's how the promoters of the fashionable, and the not-so-fashionable, diets succeed in getting you to buy their books, videos, DVDs, and food products. But here's the catch: You are likely to be losing fluid, not the fat that you want to lose.

This is where the yo-yo kicks in. Off comes the weight, a few weeks later back on it goes. Most fad diets impose major lifestyle changes and food restrictions, and these are unsustainable. The pleasure from food starts to wane, and back into the old habits you slide. Then along comes a new diet that will be the answer for you, for just $9.99, and off you go again. These popular diets can help, by giving you a kick-start. If they start you thinking about the foods that are good for you, and prompt you to start adapting your lifestyle to a healthy one, then OK. But these diets are not good long-term. Like training wheels on a bicycle, if they are there at all, they should not be there forever.

It's a straightforward equation. If weight is to remain the same, "calories in" must equal "calories out." As a rough guide, for adults performing light work, women need around 2,000 calories a day, and men need around 2,500 calories. Eat less than that and weight is lost, eat more than that and weight is put on. Reduce the number of calories you eat each day, eat less high-fat and high-sugar foods and more fruits, vegetables, and carbohydrate foods regularly during the day so you are less likely to reach for unhealthy snacks, and take part in some regular activity each day, and soon you'll succeed in your mission to lose, say, up to a pound a week. Simple, isn't it?

How do you know if you need to lose weight? What's your baseline and your goal? Check out IDEA 18, *Body mass index*, to find out.

Try another idea...

"Man lives on one quarter of what he eats. On the other three quarters lives his doctor."
INSCRIPTION ON EGYPTIAN PYRAMID, 3800 BC

Defining idea...

143

How did it go?

Q   It's tough. How can I stop slipping back into bad habits?

A   *It's often better to do it with a friend. Why not ask a friend or colleague whether they would like to lose weight with you? Be careful that they don't misinterpret this as you telling them that they need to lose weight, rather than you wanting their support. This is where weight-loss organizations can help, since for some people they provide the necessary support and motivation. Tell your family and friends that you are trying to lose weight so that they don't get offended when you decline a second portion of their speciality dessert. They can help you, too, by encouraging you and by not putting temptation in your way.*

Q   I don't want to miss out on my favorite foods. Won't life be unbearable?

A   *Moderation is the key. There's no need to exclude foods from your diet. If you do this you'll become bored eating the same old thing, and frustrated because you can't eat foods you enjoy. Before long you'll be back to where you started. That's why fad diets don't work for people. You can have fast food or some chocolate every now and then as a treat, just not every day. Try making these special foods a reward for reaching your weekly target weight loss of half a pound to a pound.*

33

Challenge cholesterol

There's been lots of talk, maybe too much talk, about cholesterol and how bad it is. But the time has come to separate the fats. Why? Because not all fats are bad.

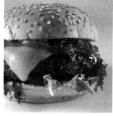

OK, let's have a quick science lesson. Fats provide energy, vitamins A, D, and E, and also the essential fatty acids that the body cannot make for itself.

Cholesterol is required for cell membrane manufacture, the production of certain hormones and to assist in the digestive process. Around 25–33 percent of the cholesterol found within our bodies comes from the food that we eat. The remainder is made in the body when fats, particularly saturated fats, are converted by the liver into cholesterol.

Sounds good so far. Now here's the kicker: Any surplus bad cholesterol (called LDL cholesterol) within the circulation may become oxidized—bombarded by free radicals, that is—and dumped on the walls of the arteries. Imagine debris collecting in a water pipe. Slowly but surely the pipe gets clogged up, hindering the efficient flow of water. This is what happens when the arteries become furred up. Blood flow is restricted, and if it becomes completely obstructed the result is a heart attack or a stroke.

Here's an idea for you... **Over the next week total up how much fat you eat. You could also get your cholesterol level checked.**

But here comes something to the rescue. There's also good cholesterol (called HDL cholesterol) that removes cholesterol from circulation.

The concern with high blood pressure is the damage it can cause to the arteries, which in turn contributes to heart attacks and strokes. Likewise, high levels of bad cholesterol, and low levels of good cholesterol, increase the risk of blood vessel damage and subsequent heart disease. So, these risk factors have a common goal. Moreover, they work as a team—or a better term would be a terrorist cell, since it's damage and death they are working toward. High levels of bad cholesterol enhance the harmful effects of the other heart disease risk factors or cell members, namely obesity, smoking, poor activity levels, high blood pressure, and stress.

So how can you reduce your cholesterol level? What's important is to reduce the total amount of fat you eat, and to change the balance of the fats you eat so that you eat less saturated fat. Most people still eat too much fat in general, more than the recommended maximum 95 grams a day for men, and maximum 70 grams a day for women. Moreover, most of the fat eaten is saturated, and it's this that increases cholesterol levels the most. On the other hand, polyunsaturated fats can lower levels of bad cholesterol but may also lower levels of good cholesterol. Monounsaturated fats, however, can lower bad cholesterol while maintaining levels of good cholesterol.

Defining idea... **"To be or not to be isn't the question. The question is how to prolong being."**
TOM ROBBINS

Put simply, reducing the amount of fat, in particular the amount of saturated fat, eaten during the day means eating less fried foods, cookies, cakes, pies, and chips, and choosing reduced-fat products when possible—low-fat cream cheese, fat-free yogurt, skim milk, low-fat crackers, for example.

You may be thinking that with these changes to your diet you may be a little short on something. Have a look at IDEA 29, _To supplement or not to supplement?_, to find out.

Try another idea...

Don't frown, here's some good news. You can eat more of the following—breakfast cereals with a high soluble fiber content, oatmeal, legumes (e.g., beans, peas, lentils), and pectin-containing fruits (citrus fruit, apples, and grapes)—these all help to lower cholesterol. Try cooking with olive oil, too.

The current target figure for cholesterol is to have a level that is less than 200 mg/dL. The target level for bad cholesterol is less than 70 mg/dL. In the future these target levels may be reduced even further. You can get your cholesterol tested by your doctor and sometimes by your local pharmacy. This can help you to see how well you are doing, and knowing your level can act as a good motivator to eat healthily.

It's not just about eating the right foods though. Regular exercise, and maintaining an ideal weight and losing some if you have to, can help to lower cholesterol levels, too.

"We cannot become what we need to be by remaining what we are."
MAX DEPREE

Defining idea...

Q Which foods have saturated fats?

A *Generally speaking saturated fats are found in foods of animal origin, particularly meat and dairy products. Saturated fat also comes from plant sources, for example palm oil and coconut oil. Some foods that contain beneficial monounsaturated fats are olive oil, rapeseed oil, avocado, and nuts.*

Q It's complicated, all these different types of fats. Can you simplify the issues?

A *It's easy to tie yourself up in knots. If it's creating problems rather than being helpful, during your next food shopping trip just try making the number of good-for-cholesterol foods—fruits, vegetables, and high-fiber foods—greater than the number of higher-fat foods in your basket.*

Q What about garlic?

A *Some research shows that garlic helps lower cholesterol. It tastes great, so why not give it a try? Use as much fresh garlic as you can in cooking and in salad dressings. Some folks even chew raw garlic cloves. Eating a diet high in soluble fiber may also help to reduce the amount of cholesterol that is absorbed from your intestine into the bloodstream.*

Q What about these foods that claim to help lower cholesterol?

A *Some new designer or functional foods—margarines and yogurts, for example—have over the past few years appeared on the shelves of food stores and claim to help lower cholesterol levels. They can help but are not a substitute for a low-fat diet, exercise, and maintaining your optimum weight.*

34

Who let the stress out?

Stress is all around. It can be good for us, and it can be bad for us. But how can you tell the difference? Let's separate the wheat from the chaff.

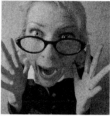

Stress, like love, is all around. You can see it and feel it but, unlike love, just hearing the word stress can make you feel bad.

You're stressed because of the amount of work you have to do; you're stressed because the credit card bill has arrived; you're stressed by your teenager wanting to stay out late and she's stressed because you don't want her to. This is how stress is perceived.

It's the long-term stress that's bad for us and this is why stress has become associated with bad news. Stress that isn't released, called chronic stress, contributes to all sorts of health problems. Stomach ulcers, irritable bowel syndrome, anxiety, and depression are some of the common ones. Long-term stress is also linked to heart disease.

Although stress doesn't cause long-term high blood pressure on its own, when you're feeling stressed you are more likely to reach for unhealthy snacks, or if you are at home, to slouch in front of the TV with a bag of chips and a beer. So long-

Here's an idea for you...

Next time you experience emotions, or feelings within your body that you recognize as being possibly stress-related, write down why you think you're feeling them. Then note down when they disappear. If they disappear once the job is done, then they are likely to be good stress. If, however, they appear for no apparent reason and seem to come and go, or are present most of the day, then they are likely to be bad stress.

term stress causes unhealthy behaviors that in turn can increase blood pressure.

Separation from a partner, death of a close family member, serious personal injury or illness, working more than forty hours a week, pregnancy or trying to get pregnant, and sexual difficulties are some of the unsurprising causes of severe stress. You may be surprised to learn that marriage or establishing a life partnership, outstanding personal achievement, and vacations can also cause high levels of stress.

But stress has been given some bad press of late. All bosses are not tyrants, all teenagers are not drug-users, and all governments are not corrupt—well, not so sure about that last one! Stress is not all bad either. Take the stress on a guitar string. Use the right amount of stress and it sounds great; too much and the string snaps. As far as the body is concerned, stress results from any change it experiences, whether it's a wanted or happy change, such as a job promotion, or whether it's an unwanted or unhappy one, such as being fired. For your body, like with the guitar string, there's good stress and there's bad stress.

We need some stress in our lives—the good stress, that is. It's what keeps us on our toes and quickens our reaction times. It helps us perform well on and off the field. You know the feeling; you're getting ready to go out on a first date with someone, or being introduced as the next speaker, or sitting waiting for the interview for the job of your dreams, and butterflies are performing circus acts in your stomach, you're mysteriously drawn to the bathroom, and your mouth feels like a monkey's armpit. Yes, we've all been there. Well, this is the effect of stress hormones—adrenaline, which gets the body charged up and ready for action, and endorphins, the body's own natural painkilling chemicals. Ever wondered why despite suffering an injury playing sports you've been able to continue? Why boxers continue through round after round of punishment? Well, that's endorphins for you. They also improve concentration and quick thinking in a crisis.

It's bad stress that we don't need. Can we do anything about it though? Yes, we can. Try IDEA 35, *Stress reaction*, to learn how to avoid the bad stress that's around us during the day.

Try another idea...

It's not just the butterflies, dry mouth, and regular bathroom trips that indicate you are feeling stressed. Constantly feeling tired all the time, flying off the handle or shedding tears at the slightest thing, having problems sleeping, not even being interested in sex, means that stress, rather than your lover, is getting on top of you. If you find that even the simplest of jobs around the house or at work are taking longer than they should, then stress may be what's getting in the way of your progress. If you are feeling like this for a lot of the time, then the stress will be harming your health.

"Without stress, there would be no life."
HANS SELYE, physician

Defining idea...

How did
it go?

Q   **I'm not the type of person that gets stressed. Why should I be interested in this?**

A   *Sorry, but it's time to stop fooling yourself. Everyone gets stressed from time to time. Feeling stressed isn't a weakness, it's a fact of life. And while you're kidding yourself that you can handle it, the stress is building up and eating away at your reserves. What happens when pressure builds up and isn't released? Things explode and go bang. It's no different in your body. Make sure that you acknowledge it and deal with it.*

Q   **The skin around my eyes gets tight from time to time, and my doctor says this is stress. Is she right?**

A   *So it's not a bad face-lift, then! Most of us have stress alert points. These are points in or around our body that our mind uses to draw our attention to the fact that we are currently feeling stressed. Most people recognize where in their body symptoms are likely to flare up. For you it's the skin around your eyes. For other people it's stomachaches and diarrhea, itchy rashes, or coming down with one cold after another.*

Q   **I always eat chocolate when I'm feeling stressed. Is there anything wrong with this?**

A   *I can see the temptation, but it may not be the best option. You just want something to cheer you up and this provides instant gratification and relief. However, these behaviors may also increase your blood pressure. Practicing relaxation techniques, doing some exercise, or having a cup of herbal chamomile tea would be better choices.*

35

Stress reaction

You can't avoid the tax man, nor can you avoid getting older. You can, however, avoid the stress that may contribute to getting your blood pressure up and bringing you down. Here's how.

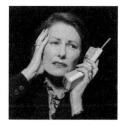

You're on your way to work, driving along your usual route. As always you reach a certain point and traffic starts to slow. Before long you are stationary.

Just like you, the steering wheel is feeling the pressure as you grip it tighter. Your jaw muscles tense, reflecting how you feel. Inside you're getting ready to explode, and before long you'll be thumping the horn. It's hardly the way you should be in charge of a car, is it? You see, stress makes us adopt bad habits, and bad habits cause our blood pressure to rise.

If you stop banging your head against the wall, the headache will go away. It's simple advice, but it's true. Likewise, if you choose another route, or another method of traveling to work, perhaps travel at a different time, your journey will be an easier, more relaxed one.

Here's an idea for you...

Take a moment to think about what causes you stress on a regular basis. Perhaps it's people trying to sell you stuff over the phone, or the fact there's never milk in the fridge at work. Now make the necessary change so that you solve the problem and avoid the stress.

Many stresses in our life are avoidable. It doesn't have to be a case of "same shit, different day." We know these stresses exist because they make us angry, irritable, fed up, on a regular, even daily, basis. They are the hurdles that get in the way of our day running smoothly. The colleague who constantly interrupts you while you're trying to work. The fact that every morning there's always a line at the station ticket office that on more than one occasion has meant you have actually missed or come close to missing your train. These are all predictable stresses. They are also minor things that shouldn't cause the trouble they do. But the fact that they keep happening means that, left unaddressed, they assume huge proportions. The fact that they are predictable is good, because you can do something about them.

If you play golf and you keep slicing your shot, you change your grip and you overcome the problem. If your cooking doesn't come out quite right, you alter the ingredients. The change is only a small one, but it can make all the difference. A gentle word in your colleague's ear explaining that you have something important to complete and need to concentrate. Buying a ticket the day before or even getting a pass so you only have to line up once a week or once a month. These are simple steps that don't take much effort but can bring you closer to the stress-free environment you crave.

The reason many of just put up with the stress, and suffer unnecessarily, is that we either believe we have no alternative or we think it'll take too much effort to change the way we behave. How many times have you said, "Oh, there's nothing I can do about it. I guess I'll just have to live with it"? Even though you may feel comfortable doing what you are doing, it's going to be causing you problems.

Often stress isn't sitting there waiting for us, it appears out of the blue. Try IDEA 36, *Stress incoming, 9 o'clock*, to see how this can be dealt with, too.

Try another idea...

Nowadays piles of paperwork are a major source of stress. These paper mountains spring up without permission. You may not be able to brush these under the carpet, but you can hide them. Not so that you forget about them, because that can cause some serious stress, believe me. But out of sight is out of mind. I know someone who had his computer in his bedroom, surrounded by piles of work-related papers. It was the last thing he saw before turning off the light and going to sleep, and the first thing he saw when he woke up. It stressed him to no end. But he solved the problem. He simply moved the computer and the paperwork to another room, leaving the bedroom for what it's supposed to be for: relaxation, sleep, and, of course, sex.

"He who rejects change is the architect of decay. The only human institution which rejects progress is the cemetery."
HAROLD WILSON

Defining idea...

How did
it go?

Q My colleague interrupts me even though I've told her I'm busy. Can you save her from a bloody and imminent death?

A   *There are a number of ways to address this problem. If your colleague is disturbing you with non-work things, you could say that you are too busy to chat at the moment and that you'd like to catch up over coffee a bit later. If it's work-related things, then ask her to list them and set a time when you can talk through them. Door open and door closed is a method of communication some people use to overcome this problem—always make sure that your colleagues understand what this means. Sometimes you just have to be firm and direct and say that you do not want to be disturbed unless it's an emergency. If you're anxious about addressing your colleague, rehearse what you are going to say first to build up your confidence.*

Q I know if I put things out of sight I'll forget to do them. Any suggestions?

A   *Try creating a "things to do box." This way you will know where the things are that need doing, but you will not be constantly seeing how large the pile is. You'll be less stressed this way, since often it's being reminded about it, particularly when you are doing something else, that causes more stress than the amount of stuff that needs your attention. By being in control and it being your choice when you look at the pile of work the stress will not be so great.*

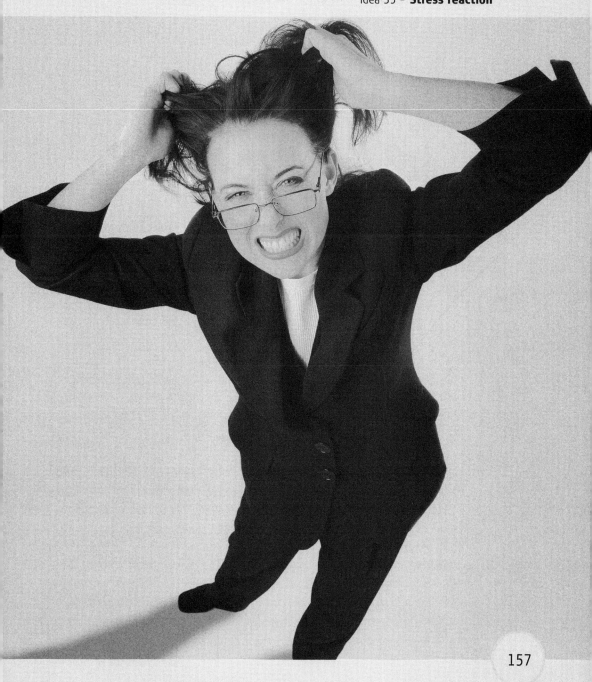

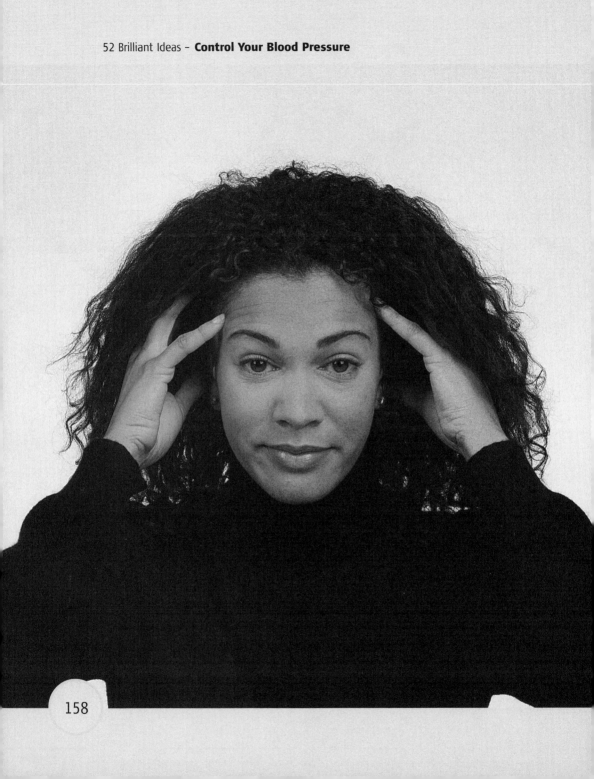

36

Stress incoming, 9 o'clock

It comes at you out of the blue. If you're lucky the problem just lands at your feet. If you're unlucky it hits you full-on in the face. Here's how to keep yourself out of the line of fire.

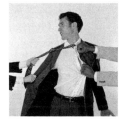

Just deal with it, will you? That's someone managing their stress, by pushing it onto someone else. Not the best way, but you can't argue that it's not effective, for them anyway.

You turn the ignition key and nothing; the battery is dead. The bank increases the interest rate on your mortgage and, bang, there goes that week in the sun. The satellite dish is installed but the roof has been damaged in the process. These things are sent to test us, and test us they do. They push our patience to the limit. They give us stress that we don't need. You can't predict this kind of stress, you certainly can't avoid it, but you can deal with it. This is where you need to reach for your immediate de-stressors.

These are simple, quick, and practical ways of taking your mind away from the stressful situation. They distract you for a moment, allowing you time to gather your thoughts so that you can turn these negative feelings into something positive.

Here's an idea for you...

Try out a few of the instant de-stressors to see which ones work best for you. Then put these around your home and your workplace, for example. Make sure they are visible so you don't have to go and search for them when they're needed.

Why do you think people advise those who are panicking or feeling under pressure to take deep breaths or to have a cup of tea? Because those remedies work.

You may see someone shrug their shoulders and say, "Shit happens" in response to this kind of stress. Well, that's one way of dealing with the situation, but this may not be enough for you. Photographs, music, muscle stretching, breathing exercises, poetry—these are all excellent de-stressors. Laughter is a fabulous de-stressor, which is why automobile organizations suggest laughing out loud rather than shouting or gesticulating like a baboon in heat when another driver cuts you off. Or would you rather have the road rage? Remember those pocket stress books? They worked on the same principle. Small and portable, they distract you for a few minutes, which is all it takes to gain control of a stressful situation.

I once attended a seminar about stress management. The speaker asked us all to say what relaxed us. The favorite things were going out to dinner, ski vacations, buying new clothes...all good but no use as instant de-stressors. You can't go skiing when stress hits you out of the blue. It's just not possible.

Everything's going fine. You've made it to the airport in good time, no delays going through security, then on the flight departure information screen a single word screams out at you. Next to your flight appears the word "delayed" or even worse, "cancelled." You want to scream back at it, you want to take that word and shove it... Anyway, that's not going to help you, is it? And neither is shouting at the first staff member you see. It's situations like this that result in the type of bad stress everyone fears. If you don't deal with this kind of stress, and let it fester, you're encouraging bad habits to develop that will cause your blood pressure to grow, too.

You are getting the hang of taking care of yourself. So now try IDEA 45, *Looking out for number one*.

Try another idea...

What you need to reach for in situations like these are your immediate de-stressors. You can use them instantly on the spot, quickly and easily. They calm the mind, they are a mental rest stop, and they calm the body, too.

It's similar with predictable stresses that you can't avoid. Financial worries, exams, the fact that you are tired of your current job and want to move on. The stress of this will become a thing of the past but it will take time for this to happen. So until that time comes, when the stress it's causing will automatically dissolve, you need to have de-stressors available. Often called coping mechanisms, they help you keep the negative stress under control and stop you from slipping into unhealthy habits, like drinking and overeating, that will raise your blood pressure.

"Success is to be measured not so much by the position that one has reached in life as by the obstacles which he has overcome."
BOOKER T. WASHINGTON

Defining idea...

161

Q   I'm absentminded. How can I remember to carry my de-stressor?

A   *One option is for you to have lots of different ones. If this is difficult for you, try singing, stretching, running in place, practicing relaxation techniques, or doing some simple yoga. Putting these into use doesn't need anything other than you.*

Q   I found that a photograph worked for a while but then it slowly stopped being effective. Should I persist with it?

A   *As soon as you notice that your de-stressor is becoming less effective, that it's taking longer for you to feel relaxed, it's time to put it on the bench for a while and introduce something new. This is why it's a good idea to have a selection of things to choose from. It's why there are so many stress toys, relaxation tapes, and so on, and why more keep coming onto the market. Don't let it stress you out that you need to change it, just do it.*

Q   I don't have any of these things to use. Should I buy some?

A   *Before you spend money on anything, take a look on your desk at work, in your car, and around your home. Anything that makes you smile, feel happy or laugh, or that brings back a happy memory will do. During the next week carry it with you wherever you go, so it needs to be quite small. When you next feel stressed take it out of your pocket or bag, hold it, and look at it.*

37

Let the mood take you

Sit down, close your eyes, and relax. Use these basics of meditation to let your mind and body unwind and recharge.

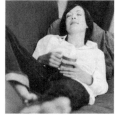

Remember the time you went on a team-building experience? Great, wasn't it? Cruising around a racetrack on a go-kart, driving 4x4s up inclines and through streams, firing paintballs at each other.

You know the kind of thing. They're a chance for you to let off steam and bond with your fellow workers. These activities serve many gods. They build camaraderie, they offer a reward for hard work, and, believe it or not, they are supposed to be relaxing.

But you don't need to leave work to achieve relaxation. In fact, you don't necessarily need to go anywhere. First of all, you need to make sure you are somewhere safe, so no driving, operating machinery, or sitting on a high stool, for example. Next, just sit down, close your eyes, and relax. These are the basics of meditation.

Here's an idea for you...

Take fifteen minutes and do absolutely nothing. Of course make sure it is safe for you to do this first. Spend 15 minutes doing nothing twice a day, every day, and wherever you like. During this time you will easily relax and unwind. You'll also learn that you do have time to do this every day and will feel better for doing it.

There's no need to panic. You don't need to hum, chant, or tie yourself up in knots. Neither will you need to undress or don unusual attire—unless you want to that is. Far from it. You're going to find out how without any physical or mental effort you can, among many others things, reduce your blood pressure. Sounds good, doesn't it? See, you are already starting to relax.

I remember my first meditation experience. I found myself at a country house on a team-building weekend. It was a Friday, the first of three days bonding with my fellow colleagues. It wasn't long after we had arrived that I was lying on the floor, eyes closed, surrounded by my colleagues, who were in the same position, being taken on a journey. First, we were instructed to find our "happy place." Next, we were led through some woods. Sunlight filtered through the trees, we felt the cool breeze on our face and leaves rustling beneath our feet, and we listened to the quiet trickle of water in the stream. It was relaxing, there's no doubt about it. In fact, I'm not a betting man but I'd wager you are feeling quite relaxed as you read this.

For some it was more relaxing than for others. As I walked through my woods I thought I heard a bear, then some giggling elves. No, I hadn't found some "special" mushrooms along the route, my colleague beside me had decided to take a nap in his woods and his snoring had made everyone start laughing. This stressed our leader, who felt we were not taking the journey seriously. He couldn't have been more wrong. The effect on us was quite the opposite. The release of pent-up energy relaxed us so well that the strength of our bonding put us at risk of never leaving that room.

Although reducing stress is said not to reduce blood pressure directly, as part of overall good health, practicing stress reduction techniques will help you avoid activities that will increase blood pressure—drinking alcohol and unhealthy snacking, for example.

Now that you are doing nothing at all, try adding to your relaxation with IDEA 41, *Handy herbs.*

Try another idea...

However, some forms of meditation can reduce blood pressure. Transcendental meditation is said to be one of the easier forms of meditation to practice. It's effortless. We like that a lot. It has good research behind it, too, supporting the fact that it can reduce blood pressure. We like that even more. And for your blood pressure to benefit, you only have to practice it for 15–20 minutes twice a day. Perfect! Basically, in it's simplest form, practitioners sit quietly with their eyes closed for around 15–20 minutes, and rather than concentrating on something, simply allow their mind and body to settle naturally on its own.

Of course, it's best to be taught how to do any form of meditation formally by a qualified instructor, but that shouldn't stop you from getting into the habit of practicing the principles.

"Life opens up opportunities to you, and you either take them or you stay afraid of taking them."
JIM CARREY

Defining idea...

How did it go?

Q   I'm too busy. How will I ever have time?

A   *If your child or a friend needed you to drop everything and help them, you would find the time, wouldn't you? So why is it any different for you to find the time for yourself? If you really don't think you can manage it, then start off with 15 minutes just once a day. You'll probably find that it's easy to find the time, and that you're more efficient as a result of it.*

Q   I tried it on the train and people kept asking me if I was all right. How can I avoid the embarrassment (and stress!) of this?

A   *This can be a problem. I grew up with a friend who studied judo. He would often be found sitting cross-legged, his hands together in his lap with his fingertips of his right hand touching those of his left. Of course, many people wanted to know what he was doing. When he said that he was looking for his chi they asked where he thought he had lost it. Those less considerate thought he was doing something he shouldn't have been doing in public. Perhaps you should try practicing the idea somewhere less conspicuous, otherwise the effects will be opposite what you want. You'll become stressed rather than relaxed.*

38

Can I have 5 minutes of your time?

Five minutes. It's not very long, is it? Time to make a cup of coffee, time to go to the bathroom. There's a lot you can achieve in five minutes. Read on and find out more.

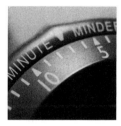

Have you noticed how it's no longer easy to estimate time? Someone wants you to do something for them and they say, "It'll only take you a minute."

I expect you've found yourself in a situation like this. If it only takes a minute, then why don't they do it?

Is it any wonder, then, that when health experts say it only takes 30 minutes of exercise a day to protect your heart you think, "Yeah right, it will take more than that, who are you trying to kid?" But it's true. Thirty minutes of moderately intensive exercise on at least five days of the week is what's recommended to protect your heart. It will also help to keep your blood pressure at a safe level. If 30 minutes seems like a long time, break it up into three 10-minute blocks, or even six 5-minute blocks. We also don't believe that a 5-minute break relaxing is long enough to do us any good. But it is.

While working spend 5 minutes every hour doing something away from your workstation that's not work-related and that you find relaxing. Read, listen to music, dance, or just make a drink. Just 5 minutes, no more, no less. The results will amaze you. You'll feel more relaxed throughout the day, and you'll still get your work completed. You may even finish it sooner so you can go home earlier. Imagine that, less time working all around.

You're bound to have heard people saying that it's important to take regular breaks throughout the working day. It's part of good stress management. If you've ever been advised to do this it would be my guess that your response would have been "I don't have time for a break." And yet, you know that very few people can concentrate for more than 45 minutes at a time. In fact, many people can't really concentrate effectively for longer than 20 minutes. Once concentration starts to fail, performance and efficiency declines, and mistakes happen. These mistakes will need to be corrected, which will probably take more than 5 minutes to do anyway.

We react negatively to the suggestion of a short break because we don't believe that 5 minutes will be 5 minutes. We've been brainwashed that it will be much longer.

Take the increasing number of cold business calls we're getting. It used to be someone from a cosmetic company ringing the doorbell. Then it was double-glazing salespeople. Now the phone is the most popular route. "Hello, I wondered whether I could talk with you. It will only take a few minutes." It never does take a few minutes, and like you, they know that. Perhaps we should time the call and when the predicted time is reached say, "Time's up. Thank you." And put the phone down.

Builders, plumbers, electricians, and the like are the same. Having asked how much and how long, there's the inevitable sucking in of breath and the pained look as he or she delivers the news. Of course the job will take longer, it always does. Multiply the time by time and a half and you won't be far out.

We're all guilty of overstretching it though. Must of us at some time would have said something like, I was up all night with the kids, or it took me forever to do it. Our gain is sympathy, and perhaps an easier day. Just 5 more minutes and we'll be home. The legendary pacifier for children in the backseat of the car.

This is why we no longer trust time estimates. Invariably the time is underestimated.

I know someone who thought he couldn't take a 5-minute break. A colleague suggested that every time he felt his mind wandering, he take a minute or two to stretch, unwind, and relax—because once the mind starts wandering it's probably time for a break anyway. All he did was get up and walk to the other side of the room and back. Then he returned to what he was doing. Before long he was in the habit of doing this without even thinking about it; it was happening automatically. The work got done, and he felt better and more relaxed throughout the day. He had a healthier lifestyle, and his blood pressure benefited.

That wasn't so bad was it? Ready for the big one? OK. Take a deep breath, sit back, and enjoy IDEA 46, *Take a day off*.

Try another idea...

"All great achievements require time."
MAYA ANGELOU

Defining idea...

How did it go?

Q   How can I remember to take these breaks?

A   *It's not easy remembering to do something when you're not used to it, when it's not part of your normal routine. Set an alarm, put a clock in front of you, ask someone to prompt you, do whatever it takes for you to grab those valuable 5 minutes each hour. Take turns with a colleague to remind each other. This way you can help each other and you will not feel guilty about taking the time.*

Q   Most of my working day is spent in meetings. How can I fit in these breaks?

A   *It may be difficult if you are in a meeting but it is still possible. Remember that most people can't concentrate effectively for longer than 45 minutes so you can use this as a reason to "take 5 everybody." Comfort breaks are acceptable and if you take the long route you'll get your break. Try setting meetings for no longer than an hour. This way you will always get the opportunity to have your 5 minutes.*

Q   I couldn't believe it. It took a week or so to get into the habit but now I'm taking 5 minutes each hour almost like clockwork. How can I convince my colleagues that these breaks won't interfere with their work?

A   *Despite taking what adds up to almost an hour off during the working day you still get the work done on time. It's no longer so scary, is it?*

39

Pet project

A dog may be man's best friend, in more ways than you realize. In fact, any pet can be your best friend when it comes to your blood pressure.

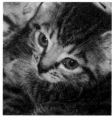

Going for a walk, chasing a stick, searching behind the sofa. Whatever you do with your particular animal it can help keep your blood pressure down.

Every year around Christmastime a message appears. It's about pets and intended for those who may not have had a pet before or who have little or no experience of animals, to make them stop and think before they rush out and buy a pet as a gift. The message reads, "A pet is not just for Christmas Day, a pet is for life." And how right they are.

A popular joke based on this message goes something like, "A pet is not just for Christmas Day. With careful planning there should be some left over for a light lunch on New Year's Day." It's funny but it highlights why the real message is necessary. No, not because people eat their pets when they're tired of them, but because many people do buy pets at Christmas or other gift-giving times of the year,

Here's an idea for you...

Spend some time every day with an animal. Spend a few minutes or as long as you like—walking, stroking, or talking to them, it really doesn't matter. Just the fact that you are spending some time on them, and on yourself, will make all the difference to your blood pressure.

often without any further thought than "I'm sure she'll love it" or "Isn't he just so cute?" Sound familiar? Of course it does. We've all been out walking and seen the fluffy little puppy out for its walk. We've probably crouched down to pet it. Maybe you've walked past the pet shop and seen the rabbits come up to the window. And what have you thought? You've thought it would be nice to have one, haven't you? I know I have.

Blood pressure is for life, too. Well, blood pressure that's at a safe level brings you a long and healthy life. Blood pressure that is higher than normal brings a shorter life, often much shorter. Your reaction to being told that your blood pressure was high and that you should do something about it was probably surprise and then shock. At first you may have buried your head in the sand, particularly if you are a man reading this, because more often than not that's what men do. It's the old "ignore it and it will go away" philosophy, which doesn't work in health. Ignore something and it invariably makes things worse. However, at some stage you probably decided to take the bull by the horns and thought, "I'm going to get on top of this." If you've only pulled your head out of the sand to read this, first of all, well done.

You're probably still frightened by the list of things your doctor advised you to do, as it can feel overwhelming.

All pets are loved, initially. The problem arises when the novelty has worn off. When the thrill of playing with this cuddly bundle of fur has gone, and all that's left is the tiresome feeding and cleaning.

You don't have to be chasing your pet around the garden to benefit your blood pressure. Take a wander to IDEA 14, *Weekend wonders,* **to see what else the outdoors has to offer.**

Try another idea...

Like pets, blood pressure needs to be cared for. The risk factors that put it up need cleaning out, the factors that keep it healthy need feeding. And this is where pets can lend a helping hand.

Whether it's a dog, cat, or even a rabbit, the pet is going to exercise you physically. The dog needs walking, the cat needs rescuing from the tree, and the rabbit often needs to be caught as it tries to escape to the vegetable patch. My parents and I spent many a happy and energetic time trying to retrieve my pet rabbit from its Xanadu that was our vegetable patch.

Any exercise is good for blood pressure. Moreover, while we are walking, rescuing, or chasing, we are less likely to eat unhealthy snacks that add to our blood pressure problems. There's actually scientific evidence to show that pets can help to lower your blood pressure. So whether it's a dog or not, a pet really can be a man's best friend.

"Walking is man's best medicine."
HIPPOCRATES

Defining idea...

173

How did it go? **Q   I don't have a pet and I'm not ready to get one. What can I do?**

A   *Find someone who has a pet, maybe an elderly neighbor who could use some help walking his dog. You could always go to your local pet store, though not every day, otherwise the staff may become a little concerned. Go every now and then. On other days just get outside, visit the country or the local zoo, anywhere where there's an opportunity to see or interact with animals.*

Q   I don't have high blood pressure. How can animals help me?

A   *If your blood pressure is at a safe level, then you want to keep it this way. It's important not to become complacent. Blood pressure can easily start creeping up into the danger zone. The theory of animals helping to lower high blood pressure also applies to keeping blood pressure at the level it should be.*

Q   Can animals help us to relax, too?

A   *Yes, they can. We like to stroke pets and when we do we feel relaxed. Even fish are relaxing. That's why you'll often see an aquarium in a doctor's waiting room. It's also why pets are allowed to visit hospitals and residential homes, for example. The mood boost we get from being around pets means we're more likely to find ourselves in the frame of mind to take on the challenges our doctor has given us to look after our blood pressure.*

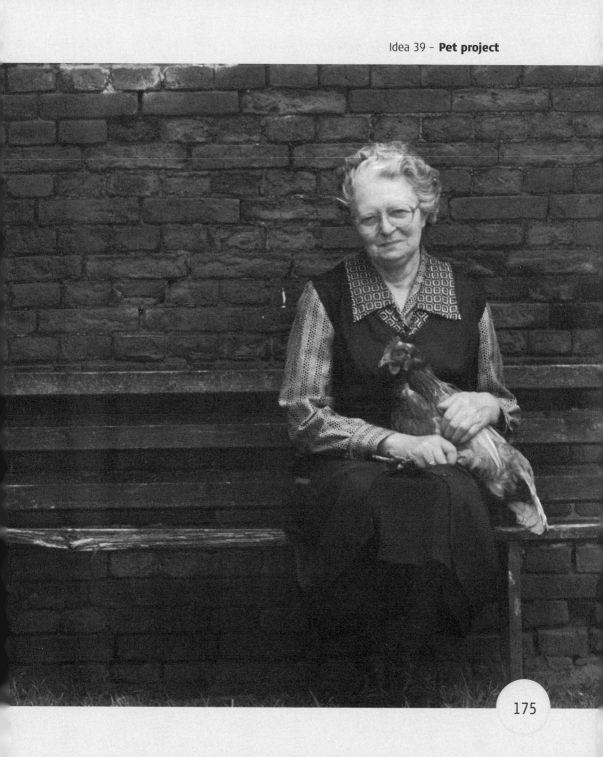

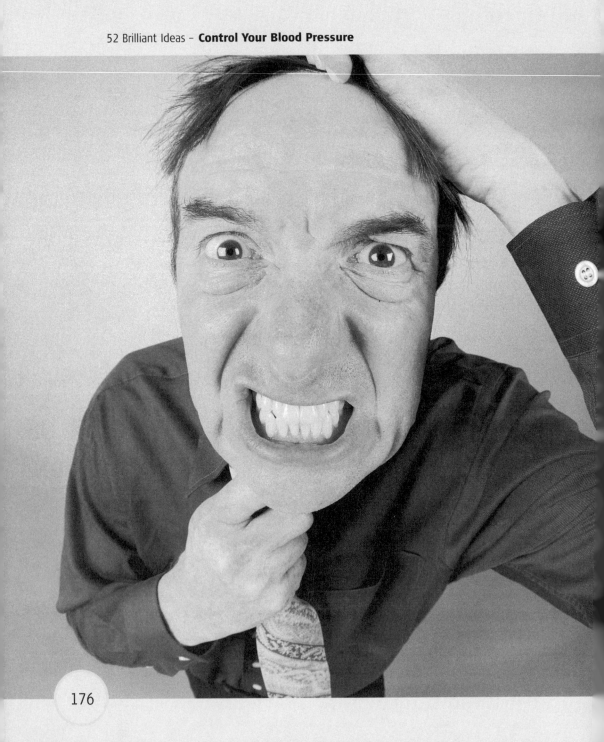

40

Bash the boss

Even if you feel like doing this when someone gets on your nerves at work there are better ways to achieve the same end. Here's how to play down work stress with toys.

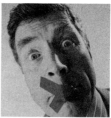

It's been a hectic week and thank goodness it's Friday. Just four more hours to go and then it's time for a well-earned couple of days off.

Your boss heads toward your office, politely asks you how you are, and then drops the bombshell. One of the company's clients wants some information, shouldn't be hard to get, it's probably best if you write it up as a report, you know what the client is like. Very sorry to drop it on you like this, I'd do it but I need to leave early today, I'm off for a long weekend. Thanks. Appreciate it.

Bang goes your weekend. Admit it, you are furious and want to kill your boss. Recognize the feeling? Of course you do. Now this isn't the best way to be. Not only might it end up with a jail term, but also, at the moment, your blood pressure is sailing upward. Kicking the desk or punching the wall isn't going to cut it. Drawing a cartoon of your boss, sticking it on the dartboard in the coffee room, and launching darts at the image may get you fired. Bashing your desk with a giant inflatable hammer, however, will calm you down.

The next time you are in a meeting or on the phone and what's being said is firing you up, start playing with your toy. You'll find that instead of the stress taking over and leading you into a shouting match, you'll be more focused on the discussion or conversation, and will come out on top.

This anger you're feeling, the tracks your fingernails are leaving in your desktop, and the mountain of stress on top of you isn't going to help you get away for the weekend. It's not going to help your blood pressure, either, if you don't do something about it.

Longer hours, tighter deadlines, job insecurity, all mean stress at work is becoming more problematic. It's one of the major causes of ill health and work absenteeism. The work–life balance is rapidly disappearing. Many companies are actively trying to reduce stress at work by offering massages, team-building retreats, and emphasizing the need for a change in work culture. But not all companies recognize stress as a problem, and you can't have an away-day each time you feel stressed. So what can you do?

Over the last few decades simple toys have been targeted at adults. Initially these went under the acceptable name of executive toys. More recently, in response to a growing need, these have been renamed as stress toys. Newton's balls were one of the earliest examples. Rubber hammers, inflatable punching bags, twisting cables, and puzzles are just some of the others. But the list is endless.

Is it any wonder they have taken off? Give a child a toy to play with and for a while at least she'll be engrossed in it. She'll sit calmly playing with the puzzle, trying to figure it out, or be happily running around chasing after the ball. The toy's material allows her to play safely, too.

Dealing with stress and playing around can use up a lot of energy. It's time for a lunch break, so have a look at IDEA 22, Lunch boxes.

Try another idea...

The role of the toys for stressed adults is just the same. They distract you from the stressful situation, pretty much instantly, and by relaxing you they keep you out of danger. For many people the touch or smell of the toy reminds them of a happy childhood memory, which instantly makes you feel good. I know someone who has a small foam ball that he squeezes in his hand when he is stressed. He also bounces the ball off the wall, and catches it, and chases it around his office. This not only relaxes him, but it also counts toward his daily activity quota. Yo-yos, slinky springs, putty, pocket pinball, or pocket billiards—with so many available there's something for everyone. The key is to get used to playing with the toy regularly, and not being afraid to do so.

"Give me a lever long enough and a fulcrum on which to place it, and I shall move the world."
ARCHIMEDES

Defining idea...

179

How did it go?

Q My colleagues keep playing with my toys and that stresses me out! What should I do?

A *Tell them to buy their own! It's stressing you out, so either hide your toys out of sight, or leave them there for coworkers to play with and get something new that's for your eyes only.*

Q I work in an open-plan office. Where can I throw my balls around (if you'll pardon the expression)?

A *You have a number of options. Take a few minutes away from the work area and go somewhere private, such as the coffee area or even the bathroom. Just find a place where you are not likely to disturb others or be disturbed. However, I know of someone who bounces around on a hop ball in and out of the partitioned office space. Not only does he relieve his stress but the amusement it brings for his colleagues helps them relieve theirs, too. You could suggest team stress-relieving breaks where you throw a foam ball to one another, so you all benefit.*

Q My toy just stresses me out more. Should I throw it away?

A *Ah, this is a very common problem. Puzzles such as the famous Rubik's Cube, computer games, and games on cell phones can have this effect. They initially start out by providing a break, which is relaxing. However, since they challenge the user this can create some degree of stress. If your toy is firing you up, it's counterproductive. Find something else, preferably something that doesn't challenge you to keep on achieving. Toys that are mindless and fun tend to work better in your situation.*

41

Handy herbs

Herbs add to the flavor of food and to the menu of good health. There are lots of ways to absorb the benefits of herbs—here's a handful of ideas for you.

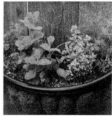

You don't often see "soap on a rope" these days. It used to be a popular stocking stuffer at Christmastime for children.

That's not to say that bathroom and other emergency presents such as candles have disappeared. Far from it. They are all over the place. Pretty collections of bath oils, soaps, and scents in cotton bags or attractive wicker baskets appear throughout the year, adapted to suit every special occasion. You may be grimacing as you recall the last time you thought, "Oh, I'll get her something for the bathroom, I'm sure she'll like that," or "He's never had a scented candle, he'll love it." But there's no need for the little pang of guilt you're probably feeling. Without knowing it you were actually helping their health. Although the current belief is that stress doesn't directly cause high blood pressure, managing stress can help you avoid the high blood pressure risk factors. There, it's fanfare time. Out of necessity has come hope, like the phoenix rising from the ashes. OK, let's not overdo it.

Here's an idea for you...

Find a gift you've put away. Some bath essence, an aromatherapy burner, a scented candle, or a pulse point herbal roller ball, for instance. Read the instructions and then use it. Over the next week use it every day. If you find more than one abandoned gift, use them on alternate days. You see, when these are used they can be very relaxing indeed.

Clever marketing has given these products a new lease on life. No longer are they just hygiene maintenance material. They have now evolved into stress relievers and are fulfilling a very necessary role.

If you're feeling a little stressed reading this, maybe because your work involves these products, then count to ten, take a deep breath, and reach for the herbs. These scented candles, bath oils, and aromatherapy burners should no longer be unwanted birthday presents that spend their lives tucked away in a cupboard. They should be welcomed with open arms.

A few drops of lavender or cedarwood oil added to a hot bath is the perfect aid to relaxation. Taking a hot soak is believed to help by convincing the body that it is now in a safe environment and that it is OK to relax. If it's safe for you to do so, then light a few scented candles and place them around the bath. There's no reason why it should only be models in TV ads who get this treatment.

Stress affects us in different ways, causing a particular part of our body to play up. It's a good idea to select the herb that helps relieve the particular symptom. If it's stomach butterflies that plague you, then peppermint or ginger would be good. If stress keeps you awake at night, then valerian, passionflower, or hops may help. Feverfew or willow bark may release the tight band of a tension headache. Be sure it's an herb you like though. Many people dislike having their

Herbs are great for dealing with stress. Take a look at IDEA 40, *Bash the boss*, to learn how stress toys help, too.

Try another idea...

clothes smelling of lavender, for example, so slipping a lavender bag into the clothes closet isn't going to help relieve stress, it's going to make it worse.

Vanilla is a smell most people find pleasant. It's one of the most popular scents, because it triggers happy memories—mother's cooking, ice cream, and holidays, for example.

Chamomile is another great herb for relaxation. It's quick and easy to use—just make a cup of chamomile herb tea. I know a woman who was finding it difficult to play her usual four rounds of golf a week. She just didn't have the energy. Her lack of energy was because she was feeling so stressed. Not able to enjoy her golf was making her more stressed. She started drinking chamomile tea a few times a day and soon was back on the course and playing better than ever. Now, it may not have been due to the chamomile alone, but it was unlikely just to have been a coincidence.

"Every action of our lives touches on some chord that will vibrate in eternity."
EDWIN HUBBEL CHAPIN, clergyman and author

Defining idea...

How did it go?

Q **I can't just drop everything in the middle of the day and have a good old soak in the bath. How can I get my herb fix?**

A *That's true. You can, however, add a few drops of lavender oil to a bowl of hot water and soak your hands in the water. If you don't have a bowl, then fill the sink and soak your hands in there. Alternatively, just place your hands under warm water from the tap and let the water flow over your hands until you feel relaxed. The sound of running water is very relaxing, too. This is a good way of relieving stress when you are at work and less disruptive than disappearing into the bathroom and screaming, which, although it may relieve your stress, is likely to stress out your colleagues.*

Q **What can I do when I'm in the middle of a stressful business meeting?**

A *Try placing a few drops of lavender onto your handkerchief. When you feel yourself becoming stressed just take your handkerchief out of your purse or pocket and sniff it. Those around you will simply think that you are blowing or wiping your nose. You could carry a pulse point herbal roller ball with you and use that. These usually contain a number of relaxing herbs and are also very discreet. You could also provide a supply of herbal teas for you and your colleagues to drink as an alternative to the usual cups of coffee and regular tea.*

42

Hairbrush idol

You may dream of a chart-topping single but you don't want chart-topping blood pressure. So grab your hairbrush and strap on your air guitar, because here's how to get yourself a platinum blood pressure reading.

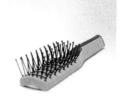

Everyone wants to be a pop star. It's not a new phenomenon. Keep on smiling in the mirror, who is it you can see?

You've strutted your stuff like Freddie, performed vocal gymnastics like Celine, and while playing air guitar assumed the position of legendary guitarists like Eric Clapton, Mark Knopfler, and Jimi Hendrix. You may be feeling a little embarrassed—oh no, somebody knows that I do it. Your dirty little secret is out. But it's not as if there's a need for an "air guitar anonymous" group. I don't know anyone who hasn't done it at some time in their life. Come on, don't tell me you haven't sung in the shower! And even if you haven't, then you most certainly have tapped your fingers on the steering wheel along to the radio.

At this very moment you are probably grinning as you think about who you would like to be. How in the privacy of your own home you've stood in front of the mirror, grasping a hairbrush, electric toothbrush, or a deodorant bottle in your hand as your substitute microphone, and sung and danced along to your favorite tunes for all you are worth.

Here's an idea for you...

Right here, right now, turn on a favorite song and sing, dance, or play air guitar to it. Or, leave the radio on and whenever a song that you really enjoy comes on take time out to sing or dance along. This is the perfect time for a break. Most songs are no longer than 3 or 4 minutes so it's not as though you will be wasting time. Do this and you'll be more focused, relaxed, and happy.

There's nothing wrong with doing it. If there were, people wouldn't take it to the next level and do karaoke. In fact, it's good for us (leaving aside the potential embarrassment of getting caught at it!). Think about how it makes you feel. It feels good, doesn't it? Just thinking about it is giving you a warm glow inside. You feel happy when you are dancing and singing, instantly you feel relaxed. You take yourself to another place for a little while, a place of dreams. It's a little escapism that distracts you from the things on your mind, the pile of work you have to do, and allows you a short break. It takes you back to happy memories. There's even more to it than relaxation. While performing vocal gymnastics or saxophone solos into your thumb you will be more physically active, too. All in all, you'll be improving your health and your blood pressure.

No one is embarrassed about entering a talent competition. Most people are proud to be able to say, "Yeah, I played in a band in college." So be proud about singing into the brush or thrashing away on that air guitar. Just don't overdo it, you don't want to dislocate anything or let your facial expression cause people to think that you need to eat more fiber!

Music therapy is a way of helping to keep the mind and body healthy. It's often used for relaxation, either through actively singing or playing an instrument, or simply through listening. It can be used to help ease pain, which is why it's played in dentists' offices and often in hospitals as well. And music is usually a vital accompaniment when doing physical exercise. Not only does it help you keep to the rhythm of an aerobic class and make it easier to do, it also helps prevent the boredom that can easily arise. You probably already know this but it's interesting to put it to the test. Next time you do any kind of physical activity, try doing the first ten minutes without music. Then switch the music on and you'll see exactly what I mean.

The music's playing, your body's moving, so now would be a good time to check out IDEA 10, *Pump that body.*

Try another idea...

A number of research studies have noted that having music playing in the background can improve a person's ability to perform tasks that require good spatial skills, such as intricate puzzles and paper folding and cutting. It also improves concentration and work performance. Depending upon the tempo, rhythm, and melody, music has the ability to arouse and calm the mind, and can lift away the symptoms of depression. It can also improve relationships. If you've ever enjoyed a slow dance then I don't need to say any more.

How did it go?

Q   I ended up listening to three songs when I should have been working. How can I avoid this distraction?

A   *It's easy to fall into this trap, especially if you are listening to an album of songs that you enjoy or listening to a radio station that invariably plays your kind of music. A way of avoiding this situation is to tune into a different station so that hopefully you will only hear songs you like every now and then. Another idea is to make a compilation tape of songs. But not the usual type of compilation tape that only includes songs you like. Make one where every other song is one that you really dislike. By doing this you'll be more likely to switch the music off after one song, rather than just going with the flow. Of course, you have to be disciplined and not hit the fast-forward button to skip past the songs you don't like!*

Q   Does it have to be pop music? I prefer classical.

A   *It doesn't really matter what type of music you listen to. It can be classical, jazz, heavy rock, or country western. Anything that you like. What is most important is that you enjoy the music you are listening to and that it makes you feel good. Ideally, it should get you moving a little and make you feel relaxed.*

43

Laugh

Laughter is the best medicine, or so they say. It's true that laughter can help keep you healthy. So go ahead, laugh. What better excuse do you need?

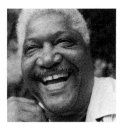

Jokes, comedians, television sitcoms, the things children say, they all make us laugh.

Everyone loves to laugh. It makes us feel good. We feel happy when we laugh.

Many TV companies have caught on to the fact that sweeping up the outtakes off the cutting room floor and sticking them together into a show makes for great entertainment. And while their viewing figures rise, our blood pressure falls.

Even when we are laughing so much that our sides are hurting, we'll keep laughing. Laughter can help to overcome pain, which is why laughter therapy is used in some hospitals. Because laughter is infectious and makes us feel good we tend to spend more time around those friends and colleagues who, by laughing, give off positive energy. This is also why it's easier to make new friends at comedy shows than at other venues.

With a little help from laughter, you can keep your blood pressure in the safety zone. By reducing stress the domino effect is that you are less likely to turn to unhealthy behaviors that increase blood pressure, such as drinking alcohol and

Here's an idea for you...

Keep anything that makes you smile or laugh handy. A joke book, cartoons, a game, even a movie—it doesn't matter. Use it every day. Give yourself a regular dose of it four or five times a day. Reach for it when you are feeling stressed and under pressure. By doing this you'll be prepared to make yourself and others laugh, and instantly you'll feel happy and stress-free.

eating sweet and salty snacks, to help you unwind. Moreover, scientific research has identified that people with a healthy heart are more likely to laugh frequently than those people who have heart disease. It isn't clearly understood how laughing helps, but it is thought that laughing may cause a reduction in stress hormones and consequently a lowering of blood pressure.

Laughing regularly and heartily can also boost your body's defenses against infection. It does this by increasing the numbers of infection fighting cells. By improving the supply of oxygen in the blood it helps healing, too.

So laughing reduces stress, strengthens the immune system, and can lower blood pressure. As Irish writer Arthur Murphy said, "Cheerfulness, sir, is the principle ingredient in the composition of health." And there's more.

Feeling a little lazy today? Not too enthusiastic about doing today's half hour of moderately intense activity? Well, here's something to help you shed the guilt and put a smile across that glum face of yours: Apparently, laughter can give you a total body workout. It's true! When you laugh your facial, abdominal, back, leg, and respiratory muscles are all worked, often quite hard. In fact, it's estimated that laughter can burn off calories that are equivalent to several minutes exercising on a rowing machine or an exercise bike. To be more precise, laughing 100 times is approximately equal to 15 minutes on an exercise bike or 10 minutes on a rowing machine. This is why you may feel exhausted after sitting in the audience at a comedy show. You thought you were just sitting there enjoying yourself when actually you had been giving your body an aerobic workout. Could exercise get any better?

Still in the mood for some fun? Spend some time checking out IDEA 17, *Get the gear*.

Try another idea...

Following the lead of Patch Adams, more doctors and nurses are recognizing the physical health benefits of laughter. Many doctors are now teaching people how to laugh to help them cope with difficult situations. Our emotions benefit from a good laugh, too. Laughter boosts mood and can help to release bottled up negative feelings such as anger and sadness. People often say that they cried with laughter, and during this they are actually laughing their negative feelings out of their bodies. By laughing we can release muscle tension and stress, and improve our concentration and ability to learn. Laughter is a tremendous icebreaker, too, helping us get along with those around us. So here's the punch line: Laughter makes life more enjoyable for everyone. And it's fun!

"The older you get, the tougher it is to lose weight, because by then your body and your fat are really good friends."
BOB HOPE

Defining idea...

How did it go?

Q **I'm becoming bored with my usual joke books. They are no longer hitting the spot for me. Should I move on?**

A *Yes, even the best jokes weaken with time. This is where the Internet is helpful. Let your friends and colleagues know that you wish to be included on the list of recipients for the jokes they send around. Be honest, it's happening so why shouldn't you be included? You could also sign up on one of the Internet sites that post jokes. Some of these sites will also send you the "joke of the day" if you request this service.*

Q **What can I do if I don't have a sense of humor?**

A *Just like everyone has a book inside them, everybody has a sense of humor. You just have to find it. Don't worry, believe it or not laughter and humor can be learned. Start by listening to recordings of funny jokes and stories. Do this for around 5 minutes a few times every day. Listen to a selection of different types of comedy, humor, and performers. This way you will find what works for you. Try reading books of jokes—not all in one sitting, but each time you take a break. Once you get home from work find a sitcom or comedy program to watch. Make your favorite cartoon, or a photograph that makes you laugh or smile, your screensaver. Or put it on your desk where you can see it easily. You could even take a class to learn how to tell jokes better.*

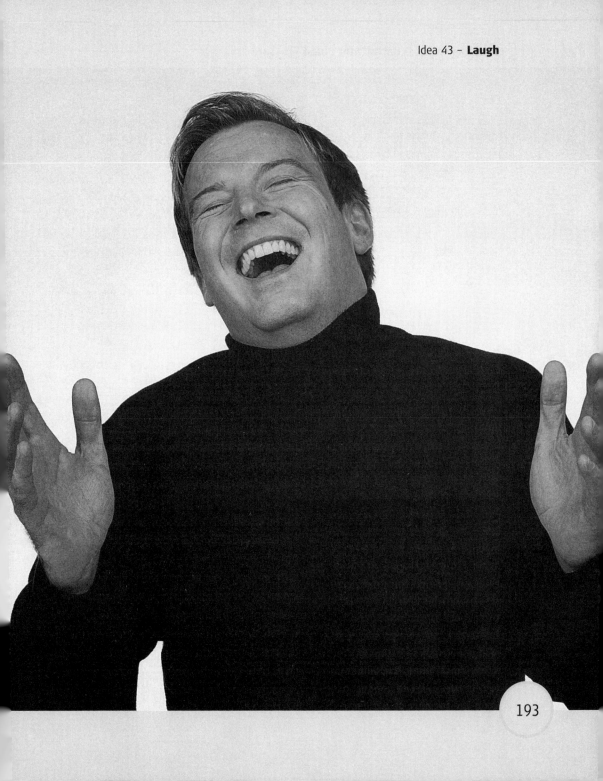

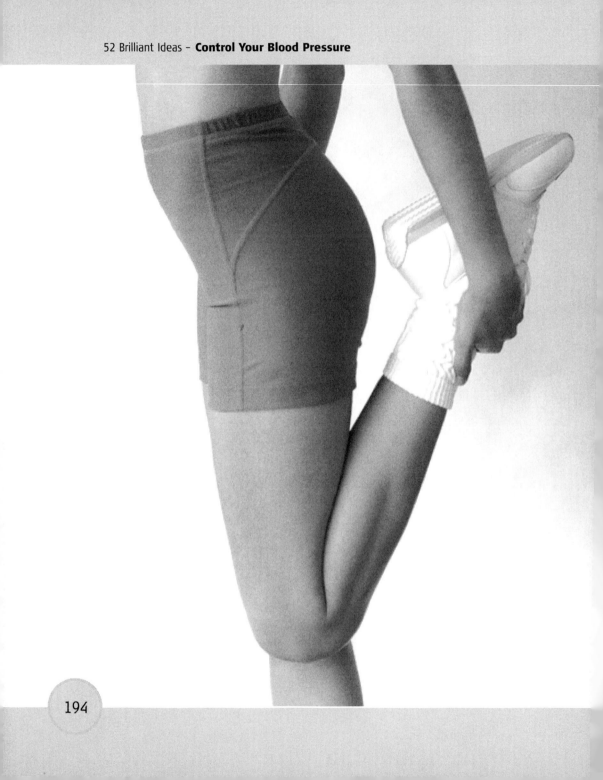

44

The joy of stretch

Anytime, anyplace, anywhere. We all enjoy a good stretch, so let's get on it.

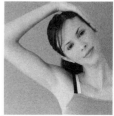

Ever felt that discomfort in your neck and shoulders? You know, when the muscles feel tight because they are knotted and, although you don't realize it at the time, your shoulders are hunched up.

That's tension you are suffering because you are not relaxed. Feeling like this means you will not be performing to your best capacity, that you will be putting pressure on other parts of your body as these try to compensate for the fact that your neck and shoulder muscles are feeling under pressure. It also means that you are more likely to reach for the cookies or chocolate, even alcohol, and that in turn will raise your blood pressure.

A good deep massage is probably what you need, but you can hardly leave your desk and spend an hour being pummeled and thumped. But all's not lost. You can help yourself with a little stretch.

Here's an idea for you...

Slowly raise your arms above your head and then interlock your fingers. Rotate your palms outward and push into the air so that your elbows are straight. Allow your arms to fall backward over your head until the first sign of resistance. Hold that position for a count of ten, and then quickly release your fingers and let your arms fall to your side. Allow them to rest at your side for a minute.

You've heard about how important it is to stretch before and after exercise. Stretching improves flexibility and helps to prevent injury. If you should fall prey to injury, stretching can aid recovery, too. Stretching may also improve physical performance. In fact, you should stretch before any intense or prolonged physical activity, even if it's decorating or moving the lawn. With so many of us spending more and more of our lives stuck staring at a monitor, we should take the opportunity to stretch while the computer boots up. (And, for once, be grateful that it takes so long…) Why? Because as you type away on the keyboard your arms, hands, and fingers are being put through an intense workout. You wouldn't jump into a workout at the gym or go for a run without stretching first, would you? So while your computer is coming to life you can bring your muscles to life, too.

Stretching is also a terrific way to instantly relax the mind and body. We do this unconsciously when we are tired. Just take a moment to think about what happens when you yawn. There's a good chance that you stretch out your arms as far as they will go. It relaxes you for bed and a good night's sleep. As you get out of bed first thing in the morning you also probably do the same thing. This time it acts to warm the muscles up for the first exercise of the day, carrying you to the bathroom or to the kitchen for breakfast. As the plane comes to a halt after a long flight you'll stretch your arms and legs as far as they will go to wake them up, too.

So go ahead, have a good stretch. You can stretch in whatever way you like, you have a free rein. Just take it gently to start with; it's easy to overdo it and end up needing the help of a physiotherapist or osteopath. Some people like to stretch their arms out away from their body as far as they can, others do the same with their legs. You can sit, stand, or lie down while you stretch, whatever feels best and comfortable, and is safe, for you.

Relaxation is also important for a good love life. With IDEA 51, *Satisfaction guaranteed*, see how blood pressure can help this, too.

Try another idea...

Here's a simple and popular stretch. Making sure it's safe—you don't want people tripping over you—lie on your back on the floor. Keeping your legs and feet together, point your toes as far away from your body as you can. Hold this for a count of ten, and then relax. You can combine this with raising your hands above your head and pushing them as far away from your body as you can.

By gently stretching you'll be achieving two things. First of all, by stretching and releasing your muscles, they will relax. Second, by focusing your attention on the stretch, you will be relaxing your mind.

"As we free our breath (through diaphragmatic breathing) we relax our emotions and let go our body tensions."
GAY HENDRICKS, psychologist and author

Defining idea...

How did it go?

Q   **It was great! But I have to spend a lot of time sitting in front of a computer. What other stretches can I do?**

A   *Place your hands together as if you are praying, holding your hands at the level of your chest. Next, keeping your palms and fingertips together, spread your fingers, just like a fan, so that your thumbs touch your chest. Slowly run your thumbs down your body until you feel a light stretch in your forearms. Hold that position for a count of ten, and then relax. You should not feel any pain while doing this, but you should feel wonderfully relaxed.*

Q   **I often get tension in my neck and shoulders, just like you described. Any tips for me?**

A   *To begin with you should ensure that you maintain good posture while at your workstation, and that the height of your chair and desk, for example, is appropriate. Next, every 15–20 minutes you should get up and take a few minutes break away from your workstation. To relieve and prevent neck and shoulder tension, try this: Using your index fingers push up your eyebrows and with your thumbs push your cheeks down. Hold for a count of ten, release, and relax. Next, slowly allow your head to sag toward your left shoulder, hold for a count of ten. Then allow your head to sag to your right shoulder and once again hold for a count of ten. Do this sequence once or twice.*

45

Looking out for number one

Unless you look after yourself you'll be of little use to yourself or anyone else. So be nice to yourself. Not sure how? Then read on. Why? Because you're worth it!

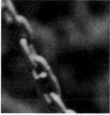

What have you done today that you enjoyed, that made you feel good? This is a question that you should be able to answer easily at the end of each day.

You shouldn't really have to stop and rack your brains for an answer. To "pass" on this question is not an option either. Not if you want to be as healthy as you can be.

I once knew someone who, when teaching junior doctors, always made sure they understood that it was just as important for them to look after themselves as it was for them to look after their patients. She used to say, "If you don't look after yourself, you can't provide the best care for your patients." It's a lesson that has remained with me for many years. It's applicable to many different walks of life— parenting, relationships, work, and your health. Basically, if you're not looking after number one, then you cannot be fulfilling your responsibilities to numbers two, three, four, etc., as well as you could be. It's simple, good old-fashioned common sense. You don't need to have a degree to understand this, but you may find that

Here's an idea for you...

Each time you do something you enjoy or that helps you, say to yourself, "I'm looking after myself." Say it as many times as it takes for you to feel happy and start smiling. You will not have to say it often. If you feel a little embarrassed saying it out loud, then say it to yourself or write it down.

you need a fairly large dose of determination and self-discipline to put it into practice.

Like many people, you probably find it difficult to put yourself first. From childhood we are taught to think about others before ourselves. In fact, should you do something for yourself, particularly if this is pleasurable, and even if those around you don't think of it as being selfish, you will probably feel a little selfish doing it. Consequently, once it's done you don't feel relaxed and happy; on the contrary, you feel guilty about what you have done. And it stays in your mind, adding more stress to an already stressful day. Sounds familiar? Sure it does.

Sadly, the next time you try to do something for yourself it's the feeling of guilt, not the pleasure, that occupies your mind. Slowly but surely you will become less inclined to enjoy yourself, and even less inclined to look after yourself because, let's face it, you feel worse afterward than you did before. Incredible, isn't it?

There's a reluctance among many people to enjoy themselves. It's almost a taboo. "She's having her hair done again," "Do you know how much he spent on that car?" Even the little things such as taking a lunch break are followed by critical comments, raised eyebrows, and tutting from those around you. It's madness because these small, but hugely self-caring, acts leave you feeling like a serial criminal.

Think about this for a moment. Over the next week at the end of each day write down something that you have enjoyed doing. Something that made you feel good. It doesn't matter what it is. What is most important is

If you really want to be kind to yourself and those around you, try IDEA 47, *It's time to quit.*

Try another idea…

that without having to think too hard you can write something down. By doing this you'll no longer feel guilty and you'll learn to accept that it's OK for you to do these things, which in fact are necessary, rather than being hedonistic.

Rather than thinking that looking after yourself and enjoying life is selfish, which it is not, think of it as self-caring. The aromatherapy massage, the night out with the guys, is a way of taking care of yourself, and of your blood pressure. It's not as formal as reducing your salt intake, which nobody will criticize you for doing because they probably view this as punishment, but enjoying yourself is still as important. Enjoyment breeds happiness and relaxation, which in turn breeds healthy behaviors that will keep your blood pressure at a level where you do not have to be worried.

"If I'd known I was gonna live this long, I'd have taken better care of myself."
EUBIE BLAKE, age 100

Defining idea…

How did it go?

Q   My colleagues at work are making comments. How can I deal with the snide remarks?

A   *You know the saying, "If you can't beat them, join them"? Well, ask them to join you when you go out for a break, or to lunch. You'll stop feeling bad, and they will start feeling good. It's a win–win situation. One of the problems with modern work culture is that it's work, work, and more work. Here's another well-known saying, "All work and no play makes Jack a dull boy." Nowadays this could be adapted to "All work and no play makes Jack a sick boy."*

Q   I'm finding it difficult. It does take determination but I still feel guilty even if all I do is take a lunch break. How can I overcome this?

A   *Incentive programs are everywhere these days. If it's not air miles that are being offered, it's points that can be used for gifts. You don't have any problem signing up for these do you? Probably not. So each time you look after yourself, give yourself a point. Let's say that you use the stairs rather than the elevator, or you eat breakfast, or you complete 30 minutes of moderately intensive activity in a day: Give yourself a point for each one. Devise your own rewards table. Perhaps three points gives you a half-hour lunch break, twenty points gives you a massage. The rewards are entirely up to you. It's the ultimate incentive program: You are being loyal to yourself. Before long you won't need the points system to reward yourself.*

46

Take a day off

Are you crazy? I don't have time. That's what you are thinking. But believe me, you do have time. It's there in front of you, so let's find it.

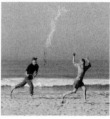

When was the last time you took a day off? I'm talking about a real day off where the only things you did were those that you wanted to do.

Not things that needed to be done like jobs around the house or in the garden, or the weekly shopping, or running the children around, or doing chores for others. A day when all you did for the whole day was enjoy yourself doing things that you wouldn't ordinarily do. Crazy things like lying in bed all day, sitting in the park reading a book with your cell phone switched off, going to watch a movie in the middle of the day and staying to watch another movie immediately after, or visiting friends or an old haunt.

We live in a world that really is 24/7. More people are now starting work earlier and leaving work later than ever before. Work pressures are crushing people into the ground. No one has time for anything anymore. Consequently, what little time comes your way is likely to be spent in ways that are not good for your blood

Here's an idea for you...

Choose a day that you would usually have off anyway, so not a workday. Put the list of things to do to one side because most to-do things can wait. Do absolutely anything you want, not need, to do. You'll see how easy it is. How you don't feel guilty after all. And most importantly, you enjoyed yourself. And you still got those to-do things done didn't you?

pressure. Down go the mugs of beer and glasses of wine, in go the burger and fries, on goes the TV. Up goes your blood pressure.

I know what you are thinking. No, I'm not a mind reader but it's many people's immediate response when they are advised to do this. However, you do have time to take a day off.

As you read this, here's what you are already doing. You are erecting barriers. You are finding reasons why you can't take a day off. You've already got things that you need to do. If you take a day off, when you return there will be even more to do. You're thinking, "No, it's simpler and less stressful not to take time off." That's why you haven't taken a vacation for so long, isn't it?

There are 24 hours in a day. Around 8 of those you spend sleeping. Take out the time spent getting up, taking a shower, eating breakfast, and whatever else you do and there's another hour gone. So in fact, a day off is only really about 15 hours. If you spend a couple of hours commuting to work each day there's only 13 hours left—since for some people this number is unlucky let's call it 12 hours that you need to take off. That's less than 10 percent of the week.

So what you need to do is to take a day off work, because you have vacation time to take but you're not taking it. It's not so difficult to do. Just look at the calendar or your planner and write "day off" across the space. Book yourself a special day where you can do something that you will really enjoy, where because you are having so much fun you will not think about work or anything else. Ideally arrange this for within the next few weeks. A day at a spa, or driving off-road vehicles, for example. It must be something that you have to pay for. If you have paid money for something, then you are more likely to see it through. It's interesting that people will happily, and easily, cancel days off they have planned that don't cost them financially, and will find excuses why they can't take the day off after all. It's the complete opposite, though, when you have had to pay good money for something—very little will prevent you from seeing it through. So by doing this you'll have a fabulous day out, you'll feel great in yourself for doing it, and you'll see how easy it was to do.

Thought I was joking in this chapter? I wasn't. But I want you to chuckle along to IDEA 43, *Laugh*.

Try another idea...

"Seize the day."
DEAD POET'S SOCIETY

Defining idea...

How did it go?

Q   It felt fantastic. When can I do it again?

A   Well done. Unless you won the lottery during your day off, then sadly I doubt you'll be able to do it every day, even though with the way you are feeling right now you might wish to. Basically, do it as often as you can. Start by getting into the habit of taking a day for yourself each week, then try taking two days for yourself every week. These two "for me" days can be separated by your usual days or taken back-to-back. Do whichever you prefer or whatever fits your responsibilities. Essentially you are making sure that you have a "weekend" each week to enjoy yourself.

Q   I'm finding it difficult. Things keep cropping up. Any more ideas?

A   OK, this is what you can do. If life keeps throwing you curveballs—for example, you are all geared up for your special day and bang, a colleague calls in sick, or your roof starts leaking and you have no choice, you have to postpone your day—just grab the bull by the horns and be spontaneous. Don't plan a day, take whatever day is available next, and have it for yourself. Aim for just one day for yourself in the next month. Or you could start by just having a half day to yourself. Then take another within the next three weeks, another within the next two weeks, and before you know it you'll be taking a day for yourself every week.

47

It's time to quit

Kick the habit, send it packing, ditch the sticks. You can call it what you will. If you've ever tried to give up smoking you know it's not easy. Here's how to make sure that with all this talk there's plenty of action.

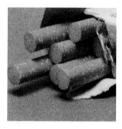

If there's one single thing that anyone can do to protect their own health, and the health of those around them, it's not to smoke. Smoking kills.

What's more, it kills people before their time, and it kills those who don't actively smoke by making them the victims of passive smoking.

OK, giving up smoking is not easy. Not for most people anyway. Sure there are some who just throw the packet of cigarettes in the trash and that's the last time they have physical contact with a cigarette. For most people who decide they want to give up though, it's very hard. Nicotine is addictive. Why else would you crave another, and another, burning stick of leaves?

Keep the receipts of the packs of cigarettes you've bought, or if you don't smoke ask someone who does smoke how many cigarettes they smoke each day. Total them at the end of the week, multiply this by 52, and then write down ten things that you'd like to have that the amount of money would pay for.

Even if you don't smoke, read on. You can relax a little and rubberneck if you like, but although you may think that you're an observer here, you still have an idea to try later on. Anyway, it doesn't hurt to understand what your smoking friends and colleagues go through.

Smoking causes a temporary rise in blood pressure but doesn't cause persistently high blood pressure. But before you use this as an excuse to light up, this doesn't mean it's OK to smoke. Smoking is very bad for your health, especially if you already have high blood pressure. Smoking damages the walls of the blood vessels, speeding up the process of hardening of the arteries that in time causes heart attacks. So smoking and high blood pressure have a common target and if you already have high blood pressure then smoking will increase your risk of heart disease and stroke even more.

Many people do not succeed in giving up the first time they try. In fact, most need more than one strike before they are out. There are some things, however, that push the odds in your favor. It's about planning and preparation.

First of all, you must have a good reason to want to give up smoking—to improve your health, to have fewer coughs or colds, to get in shape, or to save money. How many psychiatrists does it take to change a lightbulb? Just one. But the lightbulb must want to change. Setting a date is important, too. It's probably not a good idea to pick the busiest or most stressful day in your calendar. Choosing a Saturday works for many people if they don't work weekends since it's often a more relaxing day than a workday. And you need rewards to aim for, small things that you can give yourself at the end of each week you have not smoked.

After this idea you need a pat on the back so try IDEA 52, *Because you're worth it.*

Try another idea...

You also need to know how you will beat the craving for a shot of nicotine, which is where nicotine replacement therapy can help. For most people withdrawal symptoms, which many people are frightened of, usually only last for around four weeks. Smoking is a habit, too. How will you occupy your idle hands when the devil is trying to make them work? Puzzles, scribbling on paper, phoning a friend, these are just some of the things that people do to keep their hands from letting them down.

And let's not forget temptation. You need to be ready for when you find yourself in situations where you used to smoke—in the bar or after dinner, for example—all the times when you would normally light up. You know what they say about temptation? It's best to stay clear of it, until you can keep it at arm's length, that is. You could, of course, only go to places where smoking is not allowed. This way it's less likely that you'll fall victim to temptation. It's not as though you can't go without a cigarette for a period of time—if you've ever been on a long-haul flight where you cannot smoke you know you can do it.

"Defeat is not the worst of failures. Not to have tried is the true failure."
GEORGE E. WOODBERRY, poet, critic, and teacher

Defining idea...

How did it go?

Q   I don't smoke that much so I wouldn't save much money. Why should I give up this simple pleasure?

A   *You need a different motivator. Perhaps your health or the health of your children will motivate you. Do you want healthier skin or harder erections? Maybe you would like to have more energy, or to have a better sense of taste and smell. Whatever it is that does it for you, this should be your motivation.*

Q   It's hard doing it alone. Where can I turn to for help?

A   *Giving up as a solo project is certainly tough. That's why it's good to take the challenge with a friend or colleague. You can spur each other on. If you can't find anyone who wants to give up, or if all your friends are non-smokers, then get involved with a local support group.*

Q   I stop, but within a day or two I'm smoking again. What else could I try?

A   *You're not doing enough preparation. Write down the reason why you started again, the date you are going to stop, and how you are going to deal with the cravings and temptation to light up. Then give it another try. Preparing and planning is a great first step and increases the chance of successfully giving up.*

Q   I tend to smoke when I'm under pressure at work. At home I'm much less likely to smoke. Any suggestions?

A   *Find a new habit to replace smoking. A habit that is healthy, of course! Start off with simple stuff such as running in place, eating a piece of fruit, listening to music, or performing simple body stretches every time you crave a cigarette.*

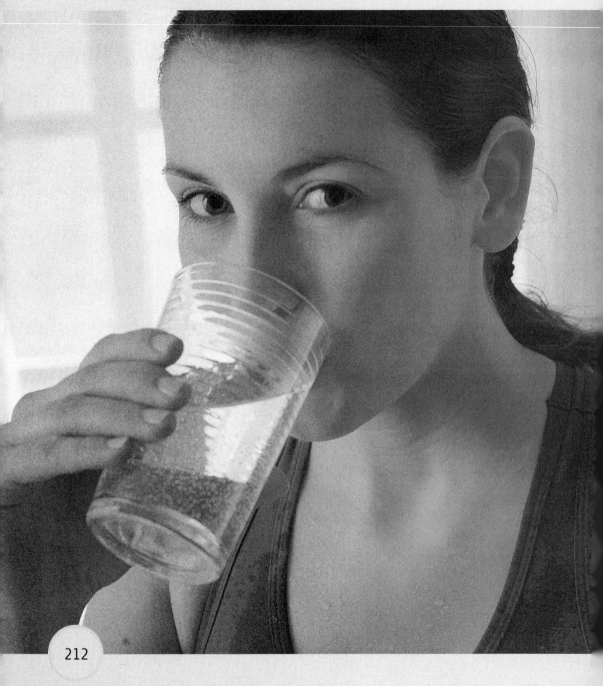

48

Water, ACE, and blockers

You take your medicine, but honestly, do you have any idea how it works? The medicine goes down, but what does it actually do inside you?

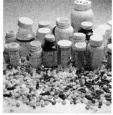

It probably came as quite a shock when you found out that you had high blood pressure. It wasn't going to beat you though. You took the advice of your doctor and followed it to the letter.

Down went your salt and alcohol intake, up went the amount of exercise you did. Hey, you even lost some weight, too.

You were looking forward to seeing your doctor again because you couldn't wait to be told how well you had done. And then your doctor's words hit you right between the eyes: "It's still too high, I suggest you start taking some medication."

Not many people want to take medication. In fact, most doctors would prefer not to prescribe it either. However, the simple fact is that many people need medication to lower their blood pressure if it is to be kept at a level that minimizes the risk of suffering heart attacks, strokes, and heart failure—and there's plenty of research to support that medication achieves this.

Here's an idea for you...

It's quiz time. Write down which type of drug is represented by each letter in the ABCD system. Also write down the names of any medicines you take and keep this list with you—it's amazing how people don't know what they are taking when asked.

Many people think that needing medication means that they have failed. It doesn't. Medication is just another helping hand. You shouldn't see medication as a quick fix, however, or as a license to live it up and let the pills do the work. You still need to address your risk factors and check them off the list. It's a team effort that's needed here, not just individual talent.

The goal is, of course, to lower your blood pressure, but how do the drugs do this? The basic principles include removing salt and water from your body, widening your arteries to enable blood to flow more easily, and making sure that your heart doesn't have to work too hard.

When doctors prescribe blood pressure lowering medication they now often use the ABCD system. Each letter corresponds to the family of drugs, for example "D" is for diuretics. The choice of drug used depends on which one is believed to be the most suitable and the best for the individual patient.

The best-known medicines for lowering blood pressure are the *diuretics*, commonly known as water pills. They flush out excess salt and water from your body through your urine. By doing this your blood pressure falls. Diuretics can also make the arteries dilate, so they become wider, making it easier for blood to flow and to flow under less pressure.

This action of widening the arteries is a common goal for a number of blood pressure medicines. A chemical called angiotensin II helps save salt and water in the body and narrows blood vessels. Now you can see that if this chemical is allowed to act unhindered the extra salt and water would be crammed into a much smaller space, pushing blood pressure up. Drugs called *ACE-inhibitors* (or angiotensin-converting enzyme inhibitors) prevent this chemical from being formed, consequently lowering blood pressure and giving the heart an easier time. Angiotensin receptor blockers work in a similar way.

Medicines can help to lower blood pressure and so can eating plenty of fruits and vegetables. How do you get enough though? Try IDEA 26, *Gimme five*, to find out.

Try another idea...

You've probably heard people talk about *beta blockers*. They slow down the heart rate. If your heart is beating too hard and too fast, then blood pressure goes up. Throw some beta blockers into the equation and your blood pressure comes down again.

And what if the muscles in the walls of your arteries become too tight? The arteries become squeezed and narrow, making it difficult for blood to flow through them easily. Again, blood pressure goes up. For the blood vessels to tighten like this, calcium needs to travel through tiny channels in the muscles. Put a block in the way, however, and calcium can't get through. And if it can't get through, your muscles won't tighten. This is how drugs called *calcium-channel blockers* work, by keeping blood vessels relaxed and open, and allowing the heart to take things easy.

There are other drugs used to lower blood pressure, but these four families are the ones that are most commonly used to treat high blood pressure.

"He that will not apply new remedies must expect new evils."
FRANCIS BACON

Defining idea...

215

How did it go?

Q I keep forgetting to take my medication. How can I remember to do this?

A   *It's a very common problem. High blood pressure usually doesn't cause symptoms, and it's often symptoms that remind us to take medicine. Think about how you remind yourself to do other things, for example, brushing your teeth. You don't need a reminder, do you? It's habit. So put your medicine next to your toothbrush—provided it's out of reach of your children. Or put your medicine near to something else that you do or use at the same time of day, again making sure it's safe to do so. If you need to take medicine more than once or twice a day, you could add this to your daily list of things to do, or set an alarm on your watch, PDA, or cell phone to remind you. Electronic cooking timers that clip to the waistband like a beeper are good for this. Or simply put the medicine somewhere safe, but where you are bound to see it throughout the day.*

Q My friends and I are all on blood pressure medication, but we are all taking different types. Why is this?

A   *Which medicines you are prescribed depends on many different things, including your age, ethnic origin, other medical conditions you may have, and medicines you may be already taking. For example, some medicines are known to be more effective for certain ethnic groups. Your doctor will have taken all these factors into account when deciding which one to prescribe you.*

49

Dump the side effects

Pros and cons, pluses and minuses, benefits and risks. This is the balance of life.

Side effects are the downside of any medication but can be overcome. Here's how.

Walking to the store, flying in an airplane, even getting out bed first thing in the morning. There's a risk of problems occurring with whatever we do, though with simple everyday activities such as these the odds are in favor of things going well and being trouble-free. Just be careful putting on your socks.

When your doctor prescribed you medication to lower your blood pressure she did so because she believed that this would benefit you. That it would lower your blood pressure so that your risk of suffering the consequences of uncontrolled high blood pressure, heart attacks, strokes, and heart failure would be minimized. You could say she was practicing damage limitation. She may, or may not, have pointed out to you the possibility of side effects with the medication. You may, or may not, have read the information leaflet that accompanied your package or bottle of pills.

The list of possible side effects on these leaflets is becoming longer. But not because there is a wider range of side effects than before. It's for legal reasons.

Here's an idea for you... **Read the information leaflet in any medication that you have in your medicine cabinet. Pay particular attention to the list of side effects and any advice given. Look to see whether there is a customer information help line. It's good to have a practice run like this so that in the future if you or friends come up against problems, like any good Cub Scout, you'll be prepared to deal with them.**

Manufacturers are required to list not only the common side effects, as they might have done in the past, but all the potential side effects, no matter how rare these might be. Important note: If you are taking medication but have not been experiencing problems and don't have any side effects, then it may not be a good idea to read the leaflet since many people, once they see the range of possible side effects, become too frightened to continue taking their medicine, no matter how many spoonfuls of sugar they are given.

Let's be honest, nothing in life is 100 percent risk-free, and if someone tells you that what they have to offer you is 100 percent risk-free, I'd be very suspicious indeed. It's the same with medicines; the bottom line is that all medication may cause side effects. It varies from individual to individual, however, and most people don't get any at all. Some get a few minor ones that disappear within two weeks of commencing the medication. For others the side effects persist and cause difficulties. It's similar to when you start a new job. You may have been confident and didn't experience any anxiety at all. You may have had a few worries for the first week or so but for no longer than that. Or it may be that months after having started you are still nervous each day. Unlike with work, however, when taking a medicine for the first time there is very little way of knowing how it will affect a person.

Based on this logic some people who need to take medication to treat their blood pressure do experience side effects. Many will just put up with them and do nothing about it, which isn't good. You didn't have any problems before you took the medicine, since usually high blood pressure doesn't cause symptoms, so why should you suffer now? To get to the root of the problem you need to do some detective work.

Since you've learned how to deal with the downside of medication, try IDEA 48, *Water, ACE, and blockers*, to learn about the upside.

Try another idea...

If you think that your medication may be causing you side effects, the first thing to do is to read the information that comes with the medication. If you cannot find the leaflet, then have a word with your pharmacist or the customer information department of your medication's manufacturer. This way you will get a good idea about whether the problems you are suffering could be related to your medicine or not.

"The healthy, the strong individual, is the one who asks for help when he needs it. Whether he has an abscess on his knee or in his soul."
RONA BARRETT, gossip columnist and entrepreneur

Defining idea...

Q I find that if I take my pills in the evening I don't get the side effects like I do when I take them in the morning. Is this normal?

A *It sounds as though you have done some good detective work and not only uncovered the problem but have also solved the crime. Usually when pills are prescribed and the instruction is to take them once a day it doesn't matter when in the day they are taken. There are some medicines, however, that although only taken once a day are best taken in the morning or at night. Just check with your doctor whether it's OK for you to continue taking your medicine in the evening. Usually what is most important is that medication is taken at a regular time each day, at a time that is convenient and that suits you best.*

Q I've checked the warnings and think my medicine is causing some side effects. What should I do now?

A *Following the logic that if you want the pain in your foot to go away you remove the stone from your shoe, you may think, "Well I'll just stop taking the medication." But although this may seem like common sense, doing this would not be very wise. So don't stop taking your medication. Remember why you are taking the medication in the first place: To lower your blood pressure. Ask your doctor to recommend an alternative for you. After all, there are lots of different treatments to choose from. By doing this you will keep you and your blood pressure safe, and you'll keep your doctor happy.*

50

Oil, water, gas, pressure—check

Taking care of your car means running through a few simple checks on a regular basis. Blood pressure is no different. So here's what needs checking.

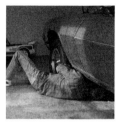

Before driving your car for any distance most automobile associations and car manufacturers recommend running through a few simple but important checks. So you do it—at least, you do it sometimes.

You do these checks because, should there be a problem, you can remedy it before the problem leaves you stranded on a freeway waiting for assistance or, worse still, is the reason why instead of driving happily in your car you are now unhappily being driven in an ambulance. It's the same reason why blood pressure should be checked, because otherwise you won't know that you have a problem until it causes you one.

Here's an idea for you...

Make a list of the tests you should have done and how often. Ask your doctor to help with this. Now check whether any are outstanding and arrange to get them done.

Before high blood pressure is confirmed it's checked several times. A single reading isn't enough since blood pressure goes up and down depending on the time of day and what you are doing. If it still isn't clear after this, then you may have your blood pressure monitored over a 24-hour period. You may have other tests, too, such as blood tests, urine tests, or an ECG (an electrical recording of your heart). They may even observe you for a few days to get a closer look at you. When these tests are performed it's to establish whether there is an underlying cause for the high blood pressure, whether it has damaged the body in any way, and to establish a baseline for future checkups.

Along life's journey—which, if you take care of yourself, should be a long and pleasurable one—regular health checks are recommended. A dental check every six months, an eye test every two years, and a blood pressure check, the frequency of which depends upon what your doctor recommends. Just like your car, your body needs regular service. This may be a small one that just involves a dipstick test of your urine, measuring your pressure, and a quick look at your bodywork if you don't have high blood pressure. Or a big one that includes everything from headlights to exhaust if you do have high blood pressure, since uncontrolled it can damage your kidneys, eyes, brain, heart, and blood vessels. The level of service you undergo, and the tests you have, will be guided by what problems may be uncovered along the way and by what has gone before.

You may or may not have noticed but each time you go to have your blood pressure checked you are asked pretty much the same questions, just like when you take your car in for service. How are you? Are you taking your medication every day? Is it causing you any problems? When did you last have blood tests taken? Make a mental note of these questions or jot them down. Next time you go, have the answers ready. This will save you some time during your consultation. If you would like to save a little more time, don't wait to be asked the questions, just rattle the answers off as one answer: "I'm feeling very well, thank you. I'm taking the medicine every day and it's not causing me any problems. Oh, and I'm up to date with my blood tests." There, you've told your doctor everything she wants to know, she's happy that you are looking after your blood pressure. All she needs to do is check it and you can be on your way to go and indulge yourself.

So you know what needs to be tested. Look at IDEA 4, *Beware the men in white coats*, to see what can happen at the doctor's office.

Try another idea...

It's helpful for you and your doctor if you have a list of the checks you should have, and how often you should have them. You may have been given a card that sets this out as a table, which allows you to check off each time you have the test performed and to fill in the results, too. This makes sure everything is checked, and by doing this you're looking after yourself and helping your doctor, who may well not have a memory of elephant-like proportions.

"A man too busy to take care of his health is like a mechanic too busy to take care of his tools."
SPANISH PROVERB

Defining idea...

How did
it go?

**Q   I have high blood pressure but haven't had my cholesterol
checked. Should I look into this?**

A   *Like high blood pressure, having a high cholesterol level is a risk factor for
heart disease and strokes. Ask your doctor whether you should have it
checked. The answer is that you probably should.*

**Q   I have the answers ready but I get so nervous that I clam up. What
can I do?**

A   *Rehearse, rehearse, and rehearse some more. Rehearse your answers in
front of the mirror or with a friend. You'll soon overcome your anxiety. It's
OK to write your answers down on a sheet of paper. Even the best public
speakers have crib notes handy.*

**Q   My doctor doesn't have a card available so I'd like to make my
own. Any tips?**

A   *Take a sheet of graph paper, or on a sheet of blank paper create the same
effect by drawing a series of vertical and horizontal lines. Across the top of
the paper write the months of the year. Down the side list the tests you
need to have done. Leave each box where the month and test intersect
blank, and block out all the remaining boxes. You should now have a chart
where each empty box represents a test and the month during which it
needs to be performed. You can create the same chart on a computer
spreadsheet, the advantage being you will not have to draw it again next
year, and you may be able to program in reminders, too.*

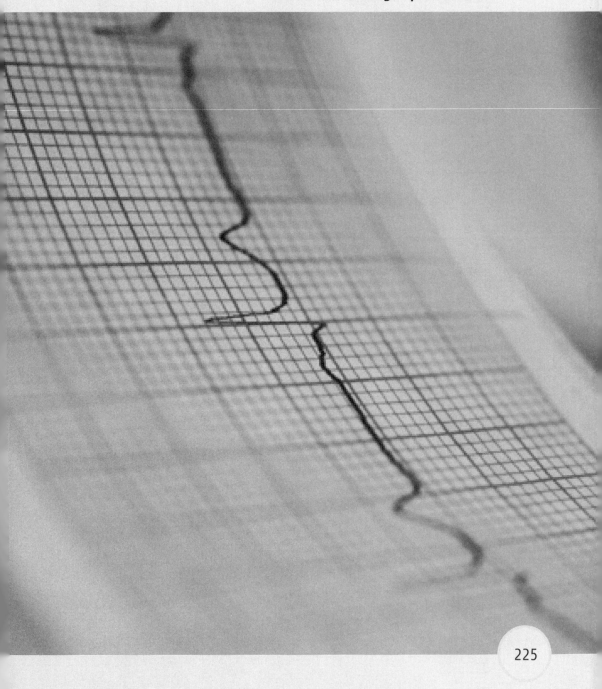

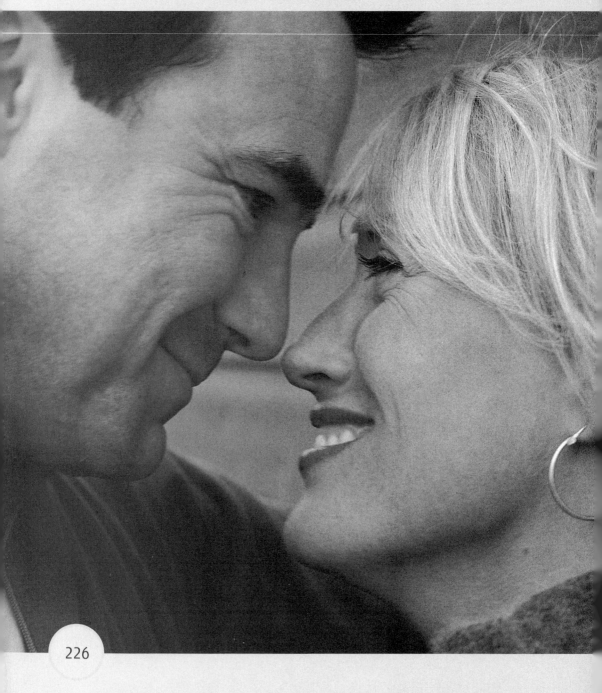

51

Satisfaction guaranteed

When blood pressure is up, a relationship may not be. A poor sex life is no joke, so dim the lights, turn on the music, and make blood pressure work for your love life.

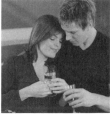

The Troggs may have sung that "love is all around" but now it's sex that's everywhere. Newspapers, television, and the Internet are full of sex and its promotion.

The flesh-filled covers of many magazines, which not so long ago would have been consigned to the top shelf of the newsstand, are now at eye level and thrusting themselves upon us. In some ways this growth of sex has left many people feeling that they are missing out, since they are not having the three-in-a-bed 24-hour sex marathons that the media would have us believe is now the norm.

You would have thought that having high blood pressure would make sex more likely. After all, for a good erection blood must fill the penis and the pressure should remain strong. But this, like many of the myths that surround sex, is a fallacy. In fact, high blood pressure makes sex less likely.

Have sex with your partner on a regular basis, as often as you like. If you're experiencing problems with erections, then ask your doctor for advice. There's no need to be embarrassed, he's heard it all before and so will be able to point you in the right direction to get the help you need.

High blood pressure can cause a man to suffer impotence, or erectile dysfunction as it is known medically, where his erection is not good enough for him to have satisfactory sex. The more his body lets him down, the less likely he is to even try.

Let's not forget the ensuing effects of this situation. It's like a line of dominoes. A man's partner may also no longer be having satisfactory sex as a result. The relationship becomes affected, with each partner believing it's their fault, or that sex is happening elsewhere. Stress increases, and unhealthy activities are used to provide some relief. These invariably add to the problem and increase the risk of blood pressure being at an unsafe level.

So it's agreed: High blood pressure can be bad for your sex life.

One area where the media is right is that most people believe that a good sex life is desirable. It's more than just being enjoyable, it may also help to keep blood pressure in the safety zone. To begin with it can be very relaxing. The right environment, food, and music all help to relax the mind. Then, of course, it's said that when done properly it's possible that every muscle in the body is worked at the same time. So it's a great way to exercise, and you know how good exercise is for blood pressure.

Sex can be exciting. So you may be thinking that this should increase blood pressure. And you would be right. Sex does raise your blood pressure, but it raises it only briefly. A temporary rise in blood pressure is normal and safe. It's part of the fight-or-flight reaction for blood pressure to temporarily go up. It goes up when we exercise. Moreover, during sex it doesn't rise to very high levels.

Sometimes it's the side effects of blood pressure lowering drugs that cause erection problems. Try IDEA 49, *Dump the side effects*, to see how to overcome them.

Try another idea...

However, it's often a case of all talk and no action. Impotence can be the first indication that a man has high blood pressure. Remember, high blood pressure doesn't usually cause symptoms. It draws attention to itself in other ways. If you or your partner are having erection problems on a regular basis—not the performance issues that often happen as a result of having too much to drink, when the most he's likely to be able to do is slur "I love you" before collapsing into a heap—then get your blood pressure checked. Do it at the local pharmacy, with your doctor or nurse, or at home with your own electronic blood pressure monitor. If you find out that you have high blood pressure this may be the first step to saving your love life, and also a step in the direction of saving your life itself.

How did it go?

Q **I feel too embarrassed to talk to my doctor about my erections. How can I raise the issue, so to speak?**

A *Most men feel the same way. Use the excuse of wanting to have your blood pressure checked to mention your erection problems to your doctor. For many men the most difficult part is getting into the doctor's office. They are frightened to make an appointment and are embarrassed about saying what's on their mind. Once you're with your doctor casually say, "I've been having difficulty getting an erection and heard that it could be caused by high blood pressure so I thought I should get it checked." Rehearse that line a few times so that you feel comfortable saying it. Now make the appointment.*

Q **I called to make a doctor's appointment and they asked me what it was for. Do I have to say?**

A *When you book the appointment you don't have to explain what it's for. If you feel you need to justify your visit, say you want your blood pressure checked. Here are a few tips to make it easier for you: You may be offered an appointment with the nurse if you ask for a blood pressure check, so emphasize that you wish to see a doctor. If you'd prefer to see a male doctor then just ask for one. And last but not least, once with the doctor mention your problem with erections right away, don't leave it until the end when there may not be enough time left. You don't want to go through all that foreplay and not fulfill your desire now, do you?*

52

Because you're worth it

The best things in life are free. Maybe. But the things that bring the most satisfaction are those we feel we deserve, that we've earned. It's time to take your reward.

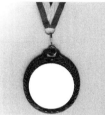

From the onset of our lives we are surrounded by rewards. Most us were rewarded for a job well done when we used the potty rather than peeing in our pants.

Clapping or approval from Mommy or Daddy was all that was needed. Now it's more likely to be bells and whistles from the potty itself. As we grew older, eating our greens would make us grow up big and strong, and if we behaved ourselves we could stay up late. Pass the school test and you can borrow the car on the weekend. Having left the security of our home, rewards became promotions, bonuses, a better car, or a bigger house.

The reward system facilitates actions that we are either in the process of learning—potty training, for example—or that we already know we should be doing but need a little encouragement to do. It's a motivator. Take smoking, for instance. If you smoke you'll be aware that it's bad for your health. As far as your health is concerned you should stop. Simple.

Here's an idea for you... **Write something you have to do on the left-hand side of a sheet of paper—a report, more exercise, for example. Draw an arrow from it to the right hand side of the page. At the head of the arrow write down something you would like as a reward for completing the task. Once the item on the left is actioned, you action the item on the right. By doing this you've made having a reward easy by making it something you must do.**

For many this just doesn't cut it, so stop-smoking campaigns have tried to be a little more specific, to hit people where it hurts. Giving up smoking will save you money, a lot of money, money you could spend on a vacation or put toward a new car. When this hasn't been enough, it's become personal. For women, the target has been their skin, since smoking prematurely ages skin and makes it wrinkly. For young men the area they worry about most has been targeted since smoking doesn't make you big or hard.

The problem with this approach is that it may not be personal enough. You may or may not have high blood pressure. Either way it's not causing you any symptoms, and sure, your doctor says that unless you keep it under control you could end up having a heart attack or a stroke. "But hey, that's not going to happen to me," you say. "I'll be fine."

We're also not very good at rewarding ourselves, and acknowledging that we've done something well. And that's the problem, learning to accept, and to be happy taking, a reward.

Let's say you want to get a massage, for the only reason that you just want one. That won't be a good enough reason and you'll need to come up with one. Something to justify to yourself and to others why you are getting a massage.

While we're on the subject of celebrating success, try IDEA 23, Bottoms up.

Try another idea...

You'll say, "I've worked really hard this week on that report, with all the hours I've put in front of the computer my neck is really giving me some trouble. I know, I'll get a massage." See how you had to find a negative, the pain in the neck, to justify it? How it should be is like this: "I've worked really hard on that report this week. I've met the deadline and my boss is delighted. I'm going to get a massage." You've done something well, so reward yourself. Of course, it doesn't have to be a massage. Your reward can be anything you want.

One way of overcoming these barriers is to think of something you have to do in the next week or so that will take some effort, that you may find a challenge, and that given the chance you'd rather not have to do. It may be something work-related like a presentation, or health-related like cutting down the amount of salt you eat each day. Once you've done this, go do something that you enjoy. It doesn't matter what it is, but afterward you'll realize how good you feel and how easy it was.

"Every day in every way, I am getting better and better."
EMILE COUE, French psychotherapist

Defining idea...

How did it go?

Q   It's taking me forever. Why do I feel I'm never going to reach my reward?

A   *It sounds like you've set the target too high. Many people do this and then often give up along the way since their reward isn't even a light at the end of the tunnel yet. Try breaking your task down into smaller, achievable chunks. For example, if you've decided that you'll get your reward once you've achieved eating five portions of fruits and vegetables a day for a week, allow yourself a reward once you've done this for four days, for example. Then have a reward after the next five days, and so on. This way not only will you get your rewards, you'll also remain positive and motivated to keep going. Once you've achieved your goal, set the next one for two weeks, then a month, so you don't stop once you've achieved the initial goal.*

Q   I don't have high blood pressure. Do I have to wait until I do before I make any changes and start rewarding myself?

A   *No. If you don't have high blood pressure, then you want to keep it this way. You still need to maintain your healthy lifestyle. If you have lifestyle behaviors that put your blood pressure at risk of becoming high, then you should use the reward system to change them, just as someone who has high blood pressure should.*

Where it's at...

52 Brilliant Ideas

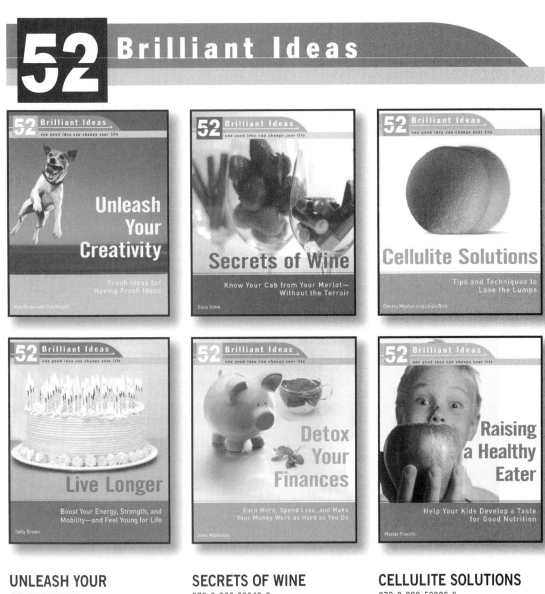

UNLEASH YOUR CREATIVITY
978-0-399-53325-9

LIVE LONGER
978-0-399-53302-0

SECRETS OF WINE
978-0-399-53348-8

DETOX YOUR FINANCES
978-0-399-53301-3

CELLULITE SOLUTIONS
978-0-399-53326-6

RAISING A HEALTHY EATER
978-0-399-53339-6

 An imprint of Penguin Group (USA)

PERIGEE

one good idea can change your life

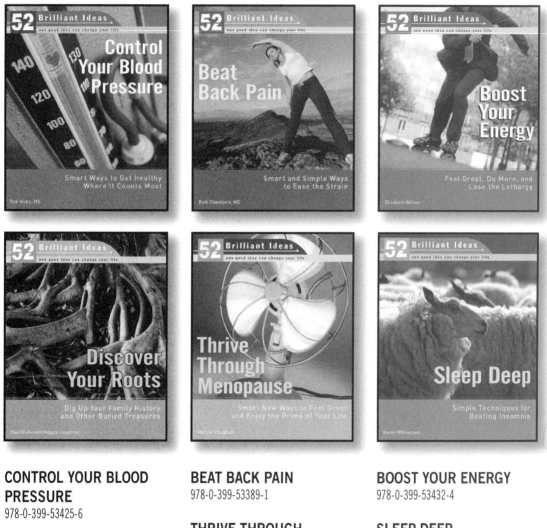